Weaning

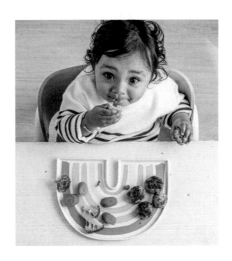

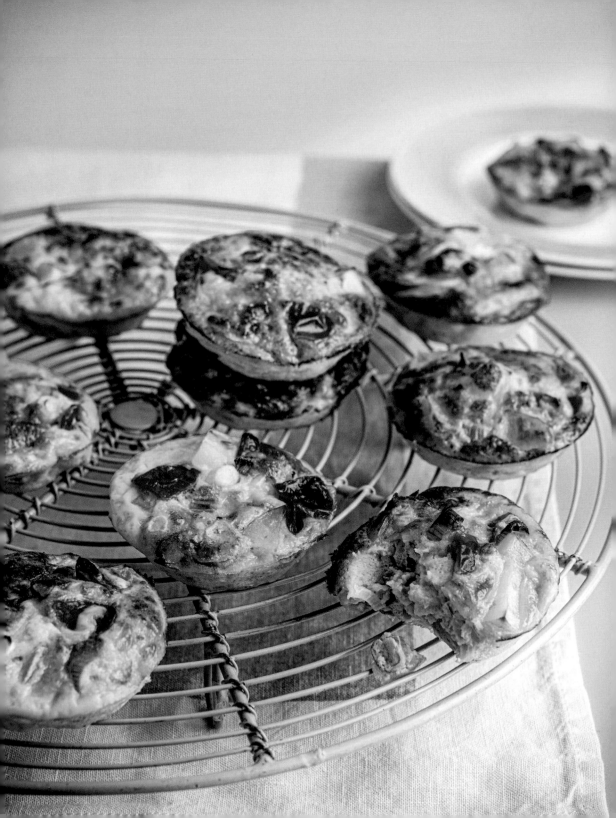

ANNABEL KARMEL

Weaning

What to feed, when to feed, and how to feed your baby

Contents

Introduction

Welcome to the wonderful world of weaning!

Weaning remains one of the biggest and often most challenging milestones in your baby's first year. There's never been so much information out there, particularly online. And coupled with the fact that babies need a nutrient-packed, varied diet from the very start to support their development, growth, and future eating habits, it can all feel overwhelming.

For more than three decades, I've guided and supported millions of families through their weaning journeys. Thankfully you've landed on my famous *Weaning* book and my jam-packed new edition has everything you need to know about your baby's food journey. Filled with nutritious and delicious recipes, meal planners, and the very latest research and advice, it's your kitchen essential.

As your baby approaches the six-month mark, they'll be going through an amazing growth spurt. Here's a fact for you; in their first year, babies triple their birth weight. They grow more rapidly in their first year than at any other time in their life. And obviously, to grow that much, they'll need a nutrient-dense diet. But that needn't feel daunting. It simply comes down to introducing a varied diet, and in this practical guide, I take you through those all-important nutrient-rich foods and how to easily include them in your baby's weaning journey.

I also explore the different ways to wean your baby: spoon-fed, baby-led, or a combined approach. Without a doubt, every method has its pros and cons. But remember, there is no one-size-fits-all when it comes to starting solid foods. It comes down to what you and your baby are comfortable with. And in this book, lots of my recipes suit whichever weaning avenue you decide to take.

What I do advocate is the introduction of soft finger foods from six months. Finger foods are the ideal way to introduce your baby to different textures, and handing over the reins to your baby has all kinds of magical benefits that I'll go on to talk about. If you're looking to nurture a little food explorer, you've come to the right place.

As with any baby milestone, weaning doesn't come without its challenges. From navigating food refusal and getting to grips with gagging and choking, to understanding allergies, I provide you with the essential information you need to wean your baby safely and confidently.

My greatest education has come from my learnings as a mom. Sadly, I lost my first child Natasha to encephalitis at three months. Although her illness was not diet-related, it became my mission to ensure that my son and two daughters were raised on the most nutritious, delicious food. I always say that I was "blessed" with three very fussy children. They led me to a career, or should I say "calling," that has seen me cook up more than 50 recipe books, produce nutritious meals for supermarkets, and curate an award-winning recipe app.

Supporting families is my mission, and I'm so pleased to have you on board. I hope that my recipes, guidance, and support provide you with the foundations for a fun weaning journey.

It's a learning curve for you both, so take it at your own pace and enjoy!

Annabel Karmel

Annabel was awarded an MBE by Queen Elizabeth II for her services to child nutrition.

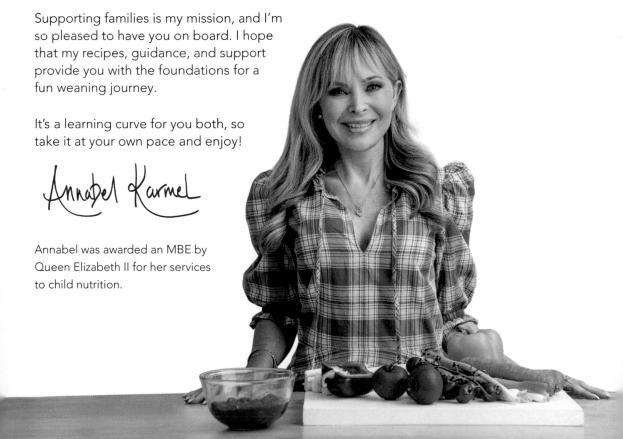

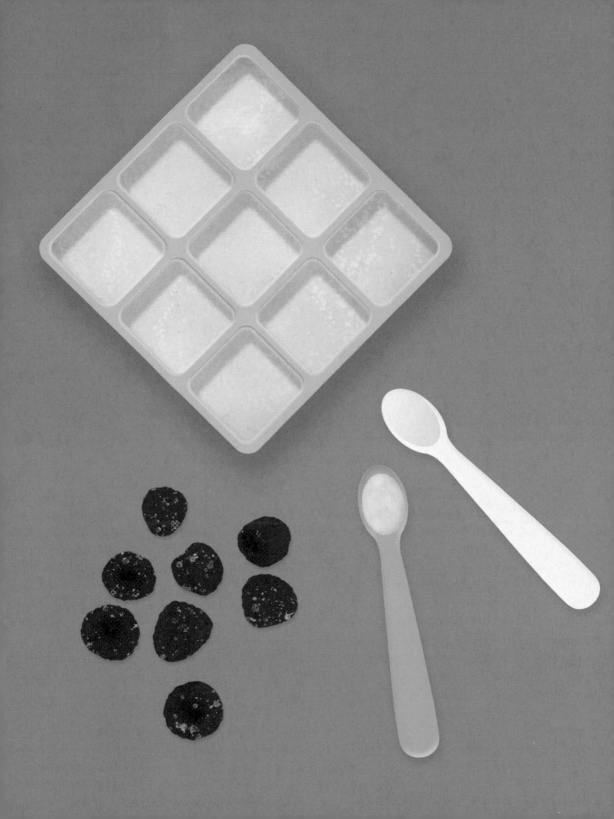

Understanding weaning

The steps involved in introducing your baby to solid food are not set in stone and you may find that she progresses more quickly or more slowly than other babies of a similar age. Some days may be better than others, too, and there will also be times when she wants only her usual milk. It helps to understand the basics of weaning and the theory behind it. Armed with knowledge, you'll be able to develop a method that works for both you and your baby.

What weaning's all about

Weaning is a gentle process that involves slowly and sensitively replacing your baby's regular milk with nutritious food that will fill her with energy and encourage optimum growth and development. Bear in mind that eating is a learned skill, like walking and talking, and will take time for your baby to master. You have a window of opportunity between 6 and 12 months when your baby will eat pretty well, so take advantage of this to introduce a variety of new flavors that should set her on a path of healthy eating for life.

Your baby's usual milk

From around six months, your baby's regular milk will no longer provide her with all the nutrients she needs—in particular, iron—and her stores start becoming depleted by this stage. This is one reason why now is the ideal time to begin weaning, as missing nutrients need to be provided by food. It is, however, very important to remember that your baby's milk will continue to form a significant part of her nutrition for many months to come, giving her the fats, carbohydrates, protein, vitamins, and minerals she needs. What's more, feeding your baby her milk will remain an important source of comfort and will help continue the bonding process.

Your baby will need breast milk or formula until she is at least 12 months old, when her diet is varied enough to offer the correct balance of nutrients. Breastfeeding can be successfully

> **"Weaning is a gentle process, involving slowly and sensitively replacing your baby's regular milk with healthy, delicious, nutritious food."**

PREMATURE BABIES

Babies born before 37 weeks will have fewer nutritional stores than full-term babies. Breastfed premature babies will require a multivitamin that contains high levels of vitamin D and an iron supplement. Some moms will also be given a supply of breast milk fortifier to enrich their breast milk. Bottle-fed premature babies will be given prescription milk fortified with vitamins and iron. A dietitian will advise when to switch to regular formula.

If your baby was born prematurely, start weaning her between 5 and 8 months after birth, but not before three months after the due date. This is to ensure she is developmentally ready to digest solids, while at the same time balancing the need for more nutrients. As with all babies, look for signs of developmental readiness (see page 27). Premature babies should be regularly reviewed by a registered dietitian who is qualified in children's nutrition.

continued alongside the introduction of solid food. There is plenty of research to suggest that breast milk continues to offer antibodies well into toddlerhood, which can help your little one resist infection. It also contains a readily absorbed form of iron, as well as protein, essential fatty acids, vitamins, minerals, and enzymes, making it a perfect complement to a healthy, varied diet.

Breastfeed your baby as usual, or, if she is on formula milk, make sure she gets at least 500 ml (2 cups) per day. Most parents find it easiest to continue with the morning and evening feeds and fit the other milk feeds around mealtimes, gradually giving a little less as their baby takes more solids. Feed your baby after her first tastes instead of before, so that she is hungrier and more willing to try the foods you are offering. Top her up with a milk feed once she's had a few spoonfuls of purée.

Introducing a mixed diet

When you begin to wean your baby, you'll be introducing her to new tastes and textures. At the outset, she'll take these in the form of a liquid purée so that it's similar to her milk— it should be almost the same consistency as yogurt—and then progress to lumpier, thicker purées, then chopped or lightly mashed. In baby-led weaning (see page 30), you'll be introducing soft finger foods.

Variety is the order of the day. Introduce your baby to new foods (including those you may not usually have yourself!) every day or so. The greater the variety, the easier it will be to progress to a healthy, nutritious diet. Small amounts represent success in the early days, so don't panic if she doesn't manage a whole bowl.

The first stage is about introducing new tastes and textures and teaching the art of eating. If she doesn't like what you are offering her today, put it aside and try see if she likes it better another day.

TOP TIPS

Before you wean your baby, it's helpful to be aware of the top tips for successful weaning:

● Make sure your baby is ready. Pushing a young, reluctant baby will make the start of weaning upsetting for you both.

● Babies sometimes find the process a little clinical and become upset when mealtimes no longer involve the comfort of sucking milk. When offering your baby her very first taste or two you may find it easier to hold her on your lap, as this will help her feel loved and secure.

● When babies feed from the breast or a bottle they instinctively push their tongue forward. Now your baby needs to learn to keep her tongue at the back of her mouth. If she can't get on with a spoon, try dipping a clean finger in the purée and let her suck your finger for the first few mouthfuls.

● Avoid feeding your baby when she's tired, irritable, or very hungry.

● Don't get hung up about portion sizes. If she's taking a little, you've done well.

● Don't compare your baby with others. She will develop at her own pace and it is no reflection on her intelligence or abilities.

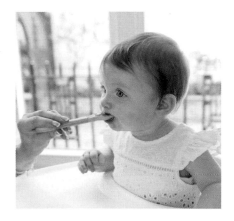

Weaning truths and myths

The process of weaning is surrounded by myths. We've got grandma telling us that babies need to be weaned at three or four months in order to sleep through the night, then reports suggesting we're giving babies a lifetime of health problems if we do it sooner than six months. So what is the truth?

Sleeping through the night
Many babies continue to wake up at night, which can be exhausting for parents. If this is the case with your little one, once the weaning process is underway make sure you give him a nutritious evening meal that contains a carbohydrate, a protein, and a vegetable. Protein takes a long time to digest and may help keep your child satisfied for longer if he is waking up due to hunger.

Teething and weaning
The development of teeth doesn't mean your baby is ready for solids. Some babies cut their first milk teeth around four months, which is early for weaning, while others show no signs of teething until well after six months.

Weight gain
It's often suggested that underweight babies benefit from early weaning; however, research shows that continuing with milk feeds helps your baby reach his optimum weight because initial foods are often low on calories.

Weaning and food allergies
Expert advice on whether the early diet of infants should include food allergens has varied over the years. However, recent research suggests that early exposure to allergens is the best way to avoid food allergies in babies. U.S Health and Human Services recommends that potential allergenic foods such as eggs or

peanuts can be introduced from six months of age. For those babies who don't have parents or siblings with allergies, or early-onset eczema, start introducing allergenic foods in the same way you would with any other food. This is because delaying introduction of these foods may increase the risk of allergies to them developing. However, if there is a high risk of food allergy (see page 18), get your baby allergy-tested before you introduce allergenic foods.

Avoiding wheat, meat, and dairy
Cutting out whole food groups is dangerous. Dairy is an important source of calcium, vital for teeth and bone growth and a good source of protein. While wheat is an allergy risk, most babies don't have problems with it (see page 22), and it is also a great source of carbohydrates, B vitamins, and fiber. After six months, it's a healthy addition to your baby's diet. As for meat, there are few other such readily available sources of easily absorbed iron.

Undigested foods
Check your baby's diaper for foods that come out whole—for example, peas and corn. This is a sign that your baby is not developmentally ready for these foods, so you need to help by chopping, mashing, or puréeing them so that the nutrients are more accessible to his body. Passing food through the digestive system is hard work and undigested foods use up energy without providing any benefit to your baby.

Critical Nutrients

As the process of weaning usually starts at around six months, it is no longer recommended that foods are introduced singly (this advice is from a time when weaning began at four months)—and giving only fruit and vegetables won't provide your baby with the critical nutrients she needs. At six months of age, it is essential to wean your baby onto a varied diet.

Breast or formula milk still supplies a lot of your baby's nutritional needs, but it's not enough for the rapid growth and brain development that occurs between now and two years of age. So what are the critical nutrients your baby needs?

Iron
Most babies are born with enough iron stored to last around six months, which is helpful as breast milk contains only a small amount of iron and the iron supplement in formula milk isn't easily absorbed. From when your baby is four months old, her body begins to use iron stores quickly due to the start of a big growth spurt. The iron is used to fuel growth and make more

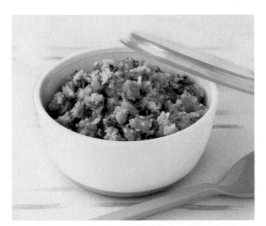

Iron-rich food. Lentils are a good source of iron and can easily be combined with nutritious vegetables.

hemoglobin in her blood, which carries oxygen to the brain, where it's needed for rapid brain development, including for intelligence.

From six months to two years, babies need more iron than at any other time in their lives. Babies who don't get enough can have sensory and cognitive impairment and it may affect their motor development. Built-in iron stores are depleted by six months—or even earlier if you were iron-deficient when pregnant or your baby had a low birth weight, so iron has to come from food. It's therefore essential to give iron-rich foods at least twice a day from six months. The best sources are red meat and dark poultry meat. Other iron-rich foods are fortified breakfast cereals; wholegrain cereal products, such as pasta; egg yolk; grains, such as lentils; tofu; dark leafy green vegetables, such as kale; and dried fruit, such as apricots and dates. Try to pair non-meat iron-rich foods with vitamin C foods as they help iron absorption.

Fats
Although adults may benefit from choosing lowfat foods, babies need higher-fat options for their health. If your baby likes fruit, serve it with full-fat yogurt and toss vegetables in melted butter. Around 50 percent of a baby's energy needs to come from fats and oils for growth and development, and a lack of fat can affect cognitive development. It won't be easy to get

FIBER

Fiber helps maintain a healthy gut and digestive system and can be found in oats, beans, pulses, vegetables, fruits, including dried, and whole grain bread. However, with foods like bread, pasta and rice, switch between white and wholegrain. Wholegrain bread, for example, is a fantastic source of fiber, but too much fiber can be a little too filling for babies. It can even inhibit their appetite and affect the absorption of key nutrients, so it's best to mix it up and let them enjoy a bit of both.

this much fat into your baby's diet because she may not eat much. Therefore it's important to choose energy-dense foods, such as whole or full-fat versions of milk, cream, yogurt, and cheese and cook with oil whenever you can. The best oils are canola and olive—high in monounsaturated fatty acids, they are good for a healthy heart.

Protein

This is the main nutrient for growth, but it can't be used efficiently by the body unless your baby has enough energy. Protein-rich foods include fish, meat, milk, cheese, nuts, eggs, beans, soy, and pulses.

Essential fatty acids (EFAs)

EFAs can't be made by the body so they have to come from food. The most important one for babies is docosahexaenoic acid (DHA), an omega-3 fatty acid, which is essential for brain development and the development of the retina. The richest sources are fatty fish, such as salmon, mackerel, sardines, and anchovies. A serving for a baby should be about 1 oz. It is important to choose fish that are lower in mercury. DHA can also be found in eggs from hens fed with omega-3-rich grains, and it does pass through breast milk. Babies who are vegan or vegetarian will need plant-based sources of omega-3-rich fatty acids such as walnuts, chia, and flax, but they may also need a supplement in order to meet their nutritional needs.

Fruit purées. These are a good source of vitamins, but from six months on your baby needs a more varied diet to ensure an adequate intake of critical nutrients.

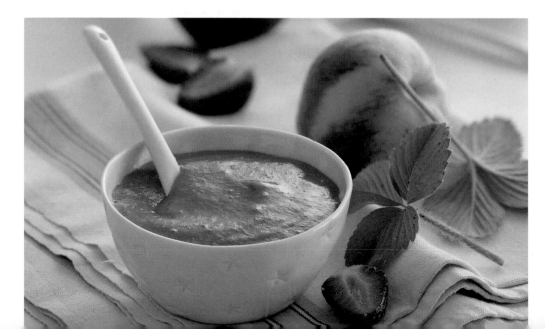

Carbohydrates

These are also energy providers and, alongside fats, provide the fuel required by your baby's body to make the best use of protein foods. Include a mixture of both white and wholegrain versions of grains, rice, bread, and pasta. Potatoes, sweet potatoes, and fortified breakfast cereals are also good sources.

Zinc

High-protein foods (see opposite) are the best source of zinc and are recommended from the outset of weaning. Zinc is needed for the development of a healthy immune system and a diet high in zinc helps to boost your baby's immunity. All of the iron-rich foods (see page 13) are also high in zinc, so if your baby has iron twice a day she'll also be getting enough zinc.

Vitamin D

This vitamin, made by the body when sunlight shines on the skin, is important for bone growth and essential for developing your baby's immune system. Fatty fish, egg yolk, and fortified foods, such as some margarines, milks, and cereals, are the only food sources we have, so your baby won't be able to consume enough.

Therefore, the recommendation is to give an 8.5–10mcg (400IU) supplement daily. Infant formula contains the supplement, but breastfed babies should receive drops (charities exist worldwide that provide free vitamin D supplements, as well as other necessary vitamin supplements, for infants).

Vitamin C

This is essential for iron absorption, healing, healthy skin and bones, and to boost immunity. All fruit and vegetables are good sources, but especially berries, papaya, mango, citrus fruits, kiwi fruit, broccoli, cauliflower, and sweet peppers.

FIRST TASTES

Your baby's first tastes are not intended to provide every known nutrient. However, because babies have small tummies, everything you serve should go some way toward helping her become strong and healthy. Babies also have fewer nutrient stores to draw from, which means that a balanced nutritional intake is important. What's more, likes and dislikes are established early, so helping your baby develop a taste for healthy foods now will make mealtimes a lot easier in years to come.

When you first introduce your baby to solid foods, portion sizes aren't important. A few spoonfuls, once a day, will give her a taste of different flavors and provide a little nutrition. In time, your baby will probably begin to eat one or two "meals" a day. "Meals" can, however, be comprised of a very small amount of food.

You'll find your baby will let you know how much she needs to eat; some foods, such as carbohydrates, will fill her more quickly than fresh fruit and vegetables. When she appears to be full, or resists your attempts to feed her, it's a good idea to stop.

By the time your baby is on three meals a day and has cut down on her milk feeds (around 7–8 months), she needs to be eating plenty of fresh fruits and vegetables, good sources of protein, healthy fats, and good-quality carbohydrates to keep her diet balanced, her body healthy, and her energy levels high. Look at her diet across the day—as long as she is getting a little of each (ideally some carbohydrate, protein, and vegetable or fruit at every meal), you are doing well.

Special diets

Whether you've chosen to remove certain foods from your baby's diet on health, religious, environmental, or ethical grounds, or his diet has to be restricted for other reasons, it's important to make sure that you make up for any shortfalls to guarantee that he's getting all the nutrients he needs.

UNDERSTANDING WEANING

Vegetarian babies

The good news is that for the first six months of your baby's life, he will get most of the vitamins, minerals, and other nutrients he needs from his regular milk. Babies weaned before six months, start off vegetarian anyway, as fruit and vegetable purées form the basis of their diets for the first month or so. Around six months is when you introduce meat, poultry, and fish, so at this time you will need to look for alternative sources of iron, protein, zinc, and vitamin B_{12} for your vegetarian baby. Vitamin B_{12} is needed for healthy red blood cells, your baby's nervous system, and healthy growth and development and you can find it in eggs and dairy produce. A shortfall can lead to anemia.

Offering dairy produce, pulses such as lentils, fortified cereals and other grains, leafy green vegetables, and fruit, including dried fruit, should help make sure your baby gets the nutrients that he needs. Provided there is no family history of allergy (see page 18), you can introduce peanut butter at this stage too. Include plenty of vegetarian sources of EFAs (see page 14), but as these are unlikely to meet his requirements, discuss with his pediatrician whether it might be necessary to top him up with a supplement.

Be aware that an adult vegetarian diet can be high in fiber, which is unsuitable for babies. High-fiber diets hinder iron absorption and are low in calories as well as essential fats, which may affect growth. If your baby is being brought up on a vegetarian diet, it's important to include nutrient-dense foods such as cheese, eggs, nut butters, and full-fat dairy products, as these will provide the extra nutrients required for healthy growth and development.

Vegan babies

If you're bringing your baby up as vegan, seek advice from a registered dietitian with expertise in children's nutrition. With careful planning, it is possible to meet his nutritional needs, as long as you always provide the critical nutrients (see pages 13–15). For protein: lentils, peas, beans, soy, and nut butters. For carbohydrates: potatoes, sweet potatoes, grains, pasta, and bread. For fats: olive oil, canola, and sunflower oil. For iron: whole-grain carbohydrates, plus peas, beans, lentils, nut butters, dried fruit, and tofu. Vitamin C-rich foods such as fruit help iron absorption.

Vegan babies may not receive adequate zinc, as phytates in food decrease absorption, and iodine can also be in short supply, so a supplement may be required. Vitamin B_{12} is found almost exclusively in animal products and so a vegan baby will only get this from breast milk (some infant formula milks are vegan but you need to make sure that you are giving correct supplements).

Vitamins and other supplements

At six months, your baby's iron stores start to become depleted and your breast milk does not provide sufficient amounts, so it is important to progress with weaning foods that are nutrient-rich and contain iron (see page 13). Discuss with your baby's pediatrician whether he should be given a multivitamin containing vitamins A, C, and D if he is breastfed.

Feeding a sick baby

When your baby is sick, follow your instincts: if he is hungry, offer him something to eat. If he shows an interest in food, stick to simple purées such as apple or banana—these place no pressure on the digestive system and they offer a little nutrition and energy. If he is not interested in solids, offer water in between usual feeds or offer more frequent milk feeds to keep him hydrated. If he is off his milk, seek advice from his pediatrician, who may recommend an oral rehydration solution. Most illnesses shift in 24 to 48 hours, but if your baby is floppy or listless with few wet diapers (signs of dehydration), see a pediatrician immediately.

Weight worries

Breastfeeding is the most effective way to prevent a baby from becoming overweight, and breastfed babies are much less likely to develop problems with obesity in later life. If you are bottlefeeding, watch how and when you feed your baby. Don't be tempted to make him finish the bottle. Look for cues that he is full, and then stop. Babies under six months old don't usually need more than 500ml (2 cups) of milk per day. Similarly, when you start introducing solids, try to avoid overfeeding him—offer tastes, and when he loses interest, stop.

If your baby is underweight, make sure he's getting enough milk and allow him to eat as much as he likes. Give a source of protein at every meal and include healthy fats (see pages 13–15) by stirring them into purées.

JENNY ASKS . . .

We plan to bring up our baby daughter as a vegetarian, but she doesn't seem to have much energy and I'm worried that her limited diet might be making her ill.

The most important thing to consider is whether your baby is getting an adequate balance of the critical nutrients (see pages 13–15).

An adequate intake of iron can be difficult to achieve in a vegetarian diet. You should include iron-rich foods two to three times a day and pair them with vitamin-C-rich food, such as fresh fruit (preferably give this after your baby's meal so she isn't too full).

Your baby should have a protein food at each meal. Good protein foods are dairy foods such as cheese, milk, and yogurt, as well as beans, pulses, and tofu. Avoid giving your baby processed meat alternatives.

If nothing seems to make a difference to your baby's energy levels, talk to her pediatrician, who will investigate this further.

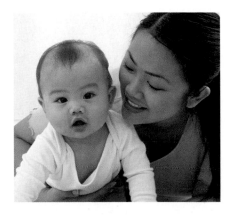

Allergy concerns

Childhood food allergies seem to be on the increase, so it's not surprising that parents are nervous about introducing foods that could cause problems. Assessing whether your baby may be at risk, and learning to recognize the signs of food allergies, can help make weaning safe and successful.

What are allergies?

A food allergy is when the immune system has an adverse reaction to a usually harmless protein, leading to the release of histamine and other chemicals that cause symptoms such as itching and swelling. Symptoms usually occur a few minutes or up to two hours after eating or can take up to 48 hours to present. Food allergies affect 3–6 percent of young children.

Specific food allergies aren't inherited, but a tendency to get allergies like hay fever, asthma, and eczema, known as atopy, is inherited from one or both parents. However, there are also environmental factors; allergies are not always inherited. To help reduce the risk of allergies, it is best to breastfeed exclusively for six months, and there is emerging evidence to suggest that introducing foods like eggs and peanuts from six months may protect a child from developing allergies (see page 12).

Top food allergies

The most common food allergens in the US are shown in the chart opposite. These must be clearly mentioned on food labels so check package ingredient lists carefully if your baby has a problem. All restaurant menus now include a standard request that you inform them of any food allergies. Some children with eczema may get a rash around their mouth when eating acidic fruit, but this can simply be a skin irritation. Other allergic reactions may range from nausea and diarrhea to rashes, and even anaphylaxis (see page 21).

Egg allergy

Being allergic to eggs is much more common in young children than in adults, but most children will outgrow it. However, children with egg allergy are also at a high risk of getting peanut and other allergies, so they should be seen by a doctor experienced in childhood allergies. Egg allergy can be to all forms of egg, but many people with egg allergy can eat baked foods containing well-cooked egg. Research has found that 70–80 percent of children with an egg allergy can eat cakes and cookies that contain egg, but in those allergic even to well-cooked egg the reactions can be severe.

A child with an egg allergy should be tested by an allergy specialist before eating foods containing egg. This may need to be done under direct medical supervision.

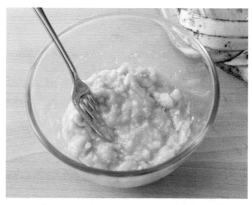

Egg replacement. Mashed banana can be used to replace egg in baking for those who have an allergy.

MOST COMMON FOOD ALLERGENS IN THE US

Cow's milk
Milk is a common ingredient in butter, cheese, cream, milk powders, and yogurt. It can also be found in foods brushed or glazed with milk, and in powdered soups and sauces.

Tree nuts
Not to be mistaken with peanuts (which are actually a legume and grown underground), this refers to nuts that grow on trees, such as cashew nuts, almonds, and hazelnuts. It is very common for foods to contain nuts.

Chicken eggs
Eggs are often found in cakes, some meat products, mayonnaise, pasta, quiche, sauces, and foods brushed or glazed with egg.

Peanuts
Peanuts are often used as an ingredient in cereal bars and in many Asian cuisines and, of course, are found in peanut butter.

Shellfish
A colloquial term for aquatic invertebrates that are used as food, both crustaceans such as shrimp, crabs, and lobster, and mollusks such as clams, mussels, scallops, and oysters, and scampi.

Sesame
Sesame seeds can be often found in bread, breadsticks, hummus, sesame oil, and tahini. They are sometimes toasted and used in salads.

Fish
Allergic reactions have been commonly reported to everything from anchovies to cod, and salmon to pollock. You might also find unexpected sources of fish in salad dressings, fish sauces, relishes, and Worcestershire sauce.

Wheat
Wheat is often found in flour, baking powder, batter, breadcrumbs, bread, cakes, couscous, pasta, pastry, sauces, soups, and fried foods.

Soy
Soy is a staple ingredient in many Asian cuisines. It can also be found in bread, desserts, ice cream, meat products, sauces, and vegetarian foods.

Some vegetables and fruit
Some produce can cause "oral allergy syndrome" or irritation of the mouth and throat. Vegetables include: celery, tomato, carrot, fennel, potato, and green pepper. Fruits include: apples, pears, cherries, peaches, plums, kiwi, and melon.

Mustard
In addition to liquid mustard, mustard powder, and mustad seeds, it can also be found in breads, curries, marinades, and sauces.

Garlic
Although garlic has many health benefits and is often used to flavor food instead of salt for babies under 1 year old, some people are allergic to it.

ALLERGY CONCERNS

EGG SUBSTITUTES

In baking, eggs can be replaced with:
- 50g (1¾oz) apple purée
- 1 small mashed banana
- 1 tablespoon of arrowroot powder and half a teaspoon of baking powder
- An additional 15g (½oz) butter and a tablespoon of water for each egg in pastry
- Self-rising flour instead of plain and 50ml (1¾fl oz) milk for each egg in cookies.

To replace eggs as a binder:
- Buttermilk
- Cornflour with sparkling water
- Chia seeds or flaxseeds mixed with water—a tablespoon of seeds to 3 tablespoons of water
- Aquafaba, which is canned chickpea liquid: a tablespoon for one egg yolk and 2 tablespoons for one egg white—this can be used to make pancakes and meringues.

Tree nut and peanut allergies

About one in 100 children in the US has a tree nut allergy, and 3 in 100 children have a peanut allergy. A child has a higher risk of developing a peanut allergy if she already has an allergic condition, such as eczema or a diagnosed food allergy, or if there is a family history of atopy, such as asthma or hay fever. Peanuts, peanut products, and tree nuts can induce a severe allergic reaction (see box, opposite), so be cautious if there is a history of allergy. In addition, there may be environmental triggers that cause an allergy.

The advice on giving nuts has changed: for babies where there are no allergy concerns, peanut butter and finely ground nuts can be introduced from six months. The advice used to be that a child allergic to peanuts should avoid nuts completely. However, there is concern that many children who do this may develop an allergy to nuts they were not allergic to because they avoided eating them at a critical time.

Tree nuts, such as cashews, pecans, walnuts, pistachios, and almonds, are not related to peanuts but can cause reactions. You may be advised not to give them if your child is allergic to peanuts. Whole nuts should be avoided until five years of age due to the risk of choking.

Cow's milk allergy

Cow's milk protein allergy (CMPA) is one of the most common childhood food allergies, estimated to affect 1.3 percent of babies aged under one. Most children grow out of it by the age of five. CMPA typically develops when cow's milk is first introduced. More rarely, it can affect babies who are exclusively breastfed, because of cow's milk protein being passed on through breast milk so you may be advised to remove all cow's milk from your diet. It will not help to switch to lactose-free products as these still contain cow's milk protein.

CMPA can cause symptoms such as eczema, wheezing, vomiting, diarrhea, constipation, hives, and/or a stuffy, itchy nose. Occasionally, it can cause anaphylaxis (see box, opposite). If your baby is diagnosed with CMPA, the pediatrician or allergy specialist will refer you to a registered dietitian.

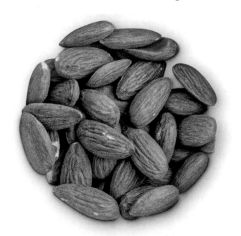

Nut allergy It is now believed that delaying giving nuts can, in fact, increase the risk of an allergy developing.

COW'S MILK SUBSTITUTE FORMULAS
Infant formula is made from cow's milk, so if your baby has a cow's milk allergy, this will need to be replaced with a special formula.
● Extensively hydrolyzed formulas and amino acid-based formulas prescribed upon recommendation by a registered dietitian.
● Soy-based infant formulas, but these are not recommended for babies under six months because of concerns about plant estrogen levels. Also around 20–30 percent of babies who are allergic to milk are also allergic to soy because the proteins appear very similar to a baby's immune system.
Note: Partially hydrolyzed formulas (available without prescription), where proteins are broken down to make them less allergenic, are not suitable for babies with CMPA.

Always consult a pediatrician or a registered dietitian with experience in children's nutrition to determine which formula is best for your baby. Early diagnosis is important because these types of formula don't taste good, but the earlier you introduce them, the more likely they are to be accepted by your baby. The dietitian will be able to suggest techniques for helping your baby transition to the new milk.

In the first year, babies will need at least 500–600ml (17–20fl oz) of hypoallergenic formula per day in order to meet their nutritional requirements.

ALTERNATIVE MILKS FOR OLDER CHILDREN
● Oat milk and milks made from foods such as nuts, soy, hemp, or coconut will not provide adequate nutrients for children under five, but can be used in cooking in place of cow's milk.
● Older children can have the milks listed above. Many of them are fortified with vitamins and minerals; a dietitian will help you determine which will best meet your child's needs.
● Rice milk is not recommended for children under four-and-a-half years old due to high

ANAPHYLAXIS
If your baby has symptoms that affect her breathing, call 911 immediately or go to your local emergency room. This is an anaphylactic reaction, which can cause a drop in blood pressure known as "shock." Symptoms include breathing problems, sudden pallor, inexplicable and sudden drowsiness, facial swelling, and possibly even collapse.

levels of naturally occurring arsenic, although rice products such as rice cake or rice pudding are fine.
Note: Sheep's, goat's, and other animal milks are not suitable alternatives for babies who are allergic to cow's milk protein as their immune systems are unable to distinguish between the protein sources—these milks will cause the same reaction as cow's milk.

If your child is fussy about having alternative milks, you will need to seek guidance from a registered dietitian who has experience in children's nutrition to ensure your child is getting the critical nutrients she needs.

MILK LADDER
Babies aged over nine months who have a mild form of milk allergy may undergo a milk challenge after following a cow's milk-free diet for a full six months.

A "milk ladder" is used to gradually introduce the milk under the supervision of a registered dietitian, starting with highly baked forms of cow's milk incorporated with certain carbohydrates and fats. If your baby is able to tolerate cooked forms of milk, she should have them routinely in her diet, in order to receive a little more calcium and other nutrients.

ALLERGY CONCERNS

Wheat allergy and celiac disease

A wheat allergy is less common and usually found in children with eczema or multiple food allergies. It is usually outgrown in childhood.

Celiac disease, which often runs in families, is different to a wheat allergy as it is an auto-immune condition triggered by a protein called gluten in certain grains (wheat, rye, barley). Symptoms include chronic diarrhea, fatigue, tummy ache, iron deficiency, faltering growth, and offensive-smelling poo. It is diagnosed by a blood test and endoscopy, but your child needs to be having wheat in her diet when tested so always see the doctor before you cut it out entirely. Unfortunately, gluten can be hidden in food such as soups, sauces, fish fingers, chicken nuggets, and salad dressings.

It's important not to cut wheat or gluten out of your child's diet unnecessarily as she may then be at risk of developing deficiencies in energy, B vitamins, and fiber.

When looking for wheat alternatives, it is vitally important to check the labeling on packaging. Gluten-free doesn't mean wheat-free. Sometimes a product may contain the rest of the wheat grain with just the gluten removed.

People with celiac disease can only eat foods labeled as "gluten-free" because even traces of gluten can cause problems. If your child has celiac disease, check food labels carefully. Don't just assume that the food is safe because even many naturally gluten-free foods can be cross-contaminated.

WHEAT SUBSTITUTES

● You can substitute wheat-free and gluten-free flours for plain flour. However, it is generally best to substitute where there is a low ratio of flour to other ingredients because then you are less reliant on gluten to hold the mixture together. Always grease and line cake tins well—gluten-free baked products tend to be more fragile.

● When you are baking, use Xanthan gum with gluten-free flour to enhance the texture so that the finished product is less crumbly.

● Crushed corn flakes or Rice Krispies make a good coating for home-made fish fingers or chicken nuggets, but not all are gluten-free so do check carefully.

● Gluten-free panko (Japanese) breadcrumbs.

● Rice flour, polenta, buckwheat, cornflour, arrowroot, and potato flour are all naturally gluten-free so are suitable for those with celiac.

● Rice noodles are a good substitute for pasta.

● Quinoa, millet, tapioca, amaranth, and rice are good alternatives to grains.

● There are many gluten-free and wheat-free breads, crackers, pasta, and pizza bases available in supermarkets.

● Cornflour and soy flour.

● Ground almonds work well in cookies, cakes, breads, and doughs.

Note: Oats do not naturally contain gluten but they are often manufactured in such a way that they can become cross-contaminated. Read the label to ensure that your oats are really "gluten-free."

KEEPING A FOOD DIARY

A good way to pinpoint problem foods is to make a note of every food you introduce, and any reactions your baby has. Even if your baby doesn't suffer from allergies, it can be useful to record details of foods she has tried. If you have allergies in the family, it is advisable to wait 48 hours between the introduction of the potentially allergenic foods to see if there is a reaction. So, try dairy produce, for example, and then wait for two days before introducing eggs. It is a good idea to introduce new foods at breakfast or lunchtime, so you can monitor your baby's reaction during the day.

FREQUENTLY ASKED QUESTIONS

Here I've addressed some of the most common questions parents ask me.

Q My husband and I have food allergies. Will my son develop them?

A No, but there is a chance he will inherit an allergic tendency, which means he could develop eczema or asthma or an allergy to something else. A tendency to get allergies and allergic problems, such as hay fever, asthma, and eczema, is known as atopy. It is more common to be atopic if both parents have this tendency. However, specific allergies are not inherited and may result from environmental factors.

Q How can I protect my baby daughter from potential food allergies?

A The best thing you can do is breastfeed exclusively for six months. There is also emerging evidence that introducing weaning foods, especially eggs and peanuts, from six months may protect against developing allergies to these foods. Avoiding particular foods during pregnancy or breastfeeding does not seem to make any difference to the likelihood of allergies.

Q Does delaying giving certain foods reduce the development of allergies?

A It is now known that delaying the introduction of allergenic foods, such as milk, eggs, and peanuts, is not helpful and can lead to a higher risk of developing a food allergy. However, if your baby has a high risk of allergy, for example she has severe eczema or there's a strong family history, then get her allergy-tested.

Q How much time should I leave between introducing each new food?

A As reactions usually happen very soon after exposure, there is no need to leave long gaps.

Just introduce one allergenic food at a time, leaving 48 hours in between each. It is important not to delay the introduction of allergenic foods as this may increase the chance of an allergy developing.

Q How do I know if my daughter has an allergy or an intolerance?

A There are two sorts of allergy: immediate onset allergies occur within minutes of the food being eaten. Delayed-onset allergies are more likely to cause your baby to have eczema, reflux, colic, or diarrhea. Intolerances are an entirely different condition, but can be just as upsetting. If your baby is suffering from any unusual symptoms after eating particular foods, it's important that you take her to see her pediatrician and meanwhile withhold the offending food. If you are unable to identify this, you can ask for a referral to a registered dietitian with expertise in children's nutrition, who can guide you through an elimination diet.

Q How much of an allergen is needed to trigger an allergic response?

A Immediate-onset allergies can be caused by a very small exposure to an allergen, although severe reactions will not happen unless the food is eaten. Contact with the skin will only cause minor reactions. With delayed-onset reactions, where a food such as milk or soy causes chronic symptoms such as eczema, reflux, or colic, it will be worse the more of the allergen that is consumed.

Q How do I arrange for my daughter to have an allergy test?

A If you are concerned about food allergies, ask your pediatrician for a referral to a local allergy specialist for allergy testing. Don't buy allergy tests from the internet because they are unreliable and often lead to misdiagnosis. Allergy tests can be arranged privately if there is a long waiting list—again, your pediatrician will refer you.

Q How do I arrange for my child to see a registered dietitian?

A Your child's pediatrician can make a referral to a registered dietitian with expertise in children's nutrition. You can also self-refer to a registered dietitian at a private practice, but make sure you find one who has expertise in children's nutrition.

Q If my baby is allergic to one food, is she likely to have other food allergies?

A Babies who have eczema and particularly those who developed eczema early in life, especially in the first three to four months, are more likely to develop an allergy. Having another type of food allergy, also increases the risk. For example, babies and children with an egg allergy are at a high risk of developing a peanut allergy, so they should always be seen by a specialist experienced in childhood allergies.

Q Will my baby outgrow his allergy?

A Fortunately, allergies to milk, egg, soy, and wheat are usually outgrown during childhood, while allergies to peanut, tree nuts, fish, and shellfish tend to persist into adulthood.

Q My son has a severe peanut allergy. Will my baby daughter also get it?

A If your baby has a sibling or a parent with a history of food allergy, then there is a good chance that they will inherit an allergic tendency, which means they could develop eczema or asthma or an allergy to something else. However, specific allergies are not inherited. Consider getting your baby tested just before weaning so that if the test is negative, peanuts can be introduced into their diet, to reduce the risk of an allergy to it developing.

Q What are the links between asthma, eczema, and allergies?

A These are all atopic diseases, meaning that they are all related to allergies. Children who are atopic (the inherited tendency to get allergies) often go through the "allergic march"—a progression of conditions. This usually starts with eczema in infancy, which predisposes to getting food allergies. Both these conditions often improve, but give way to respiratory allergy including asthma and hay fever.

Q My son is allergic to dairy. When can I start to reintroduce cow's milk?

A This is dependent upon the symptoms. It will be decided by a registered dietitian who follows official guidelines managing milk allergy.

Q I'm still breastfeeding. If my son has a food allergy, do I need to cut that food out of my diet?

A If your baby is allergic to certain foods such as milk, egg, soy, or wheat, what you eat can sometimes pass via your breast milk into their diet, although it is rare. Rather than having an immediate reaction, there may be a delayed reaction, affecting the gut or a worsening of eczema, for example. You should seek advice before trying to cut any foods out of your own diet. For example, if you cut milk from your diet, you will need to include an alternative source of protein and calcium to make sure that your milk is providing enough calcium for your baby. In this instance I would suggest seeing a registered dietitian with expertise in children's nutrition.

Q What is a food challenge?

A Apart from a skin prick test or blood test, one of the best ways to diagnose a food allergy is a food challenge. The child is put on an elimination diet where the suspected food or foods are removed from the diet, then reintroduced under medical supervision and the child is watched for signs and symptoms of an allergic reaction.

Reflux, constipation, and diarrhea

Gastrointestinal and bowel problems can be an unfortunate side-effect of many allergy-related conditions. Look out for the signs and symptoms and don't hesitate to seek advice from your child's pediatrician if you have any concerns.

Gastroesophageal reflux

Gastroesophageal reflux is a condition in which the stomach contents—food (milk) and acid—come back up into the esophagus (food pipe) or into the mouth. This condition can sometimes be a sign of cow's milk protein allergy (see page 20).

Most babies have a degree of reflux because the muscular valve at the end of their esophagus, which acts to keep food in the stomach, hasn't developed fully yet. This means that when your baby's stomach is full, milk can come back up. If he brings up small amounts of milk it's called spitting up and this is normal. Babies often spit up a bit when burping, hence the use of muslin burp clothes over the shoulder.

During a baby's first year, the muscular valve gradually gets stronger and better at keeping food down, so the spitting up reduces and the chance of having reflux decreases. It's only when strong acid from the baby's stomach comes up into his esophagus that it can be painful and start to cause problems—this is called gastroesophageal reflux and is not that common.

Around 50 percent of all babies will experience some reflux during their first three months, but this will prove to be a problem for only a very few and they will usually outgrow it. By the age of 10 months, the number of babies experiencing reflux will have dropped to around 5 percent.

Symptoms of reflux

If your baby shows discomfort when feeding, such as arching his back, refusing to feed, and crying, it can be a sign of reflux. He may also frequently vomit or spit up more than normal (spitting up is only about a teaspoon) and cough a lot, including at night, with no other sign of a cold. Other symptoms include excessive regurgitation, weight loss or poor weight gain, and waking often. To alleviate the symptoms of reflux:

- Give small frequent feeds (6–7 feeds a day).
- Avoid the slump position, which adds pressure to the stomach—this can happen when a baby is seated in a bouncy chair or car seat.
- Try to keep your baby upright during feeding and for about 20 minutes after.
- In more severe cases, your pediatrician or dietitian may suggest adding infant antacid to your baby's formula or expressed breast milk. Note that infant antacid is a completely different product from antacid. Only use feed thickeners and thickened milk if advised to do so by your pediatrician or dietitian.

Constipation

Sometimes babies become constipated when they are first introduced to solids after being exclusively breastfed. It can also be caused by not eating enough fiber-rich foods such as vegetables, fruit, and wholegrain cereals or not drinking enough fluids. You can try to stimulate your baby's bowels by bicycling his legs around

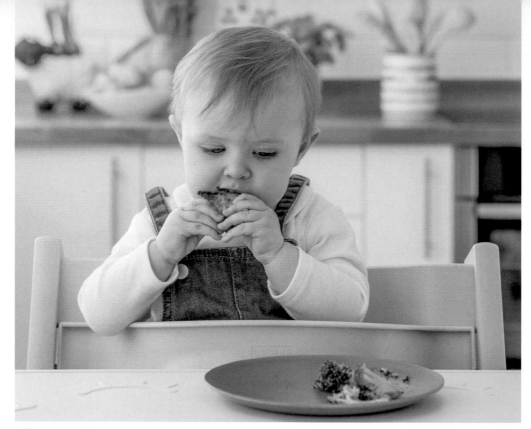

A fiber boost. Giving your baby foods rich in soluble fiber can help relieve constipation.

while he lies on his back or gently massaging his tummy. Foods that can help relieve constipation are those that contain soluble fiber (see page 14). Don't give bran or bran-containing products as this is insoluble fiber, which a baby's bowels are not mature enough to deal with.

Diarrhea

Diarrhea is when the poo is watery and offensive-smelling. In babies, frequent abnormal watery stools are often caused by a viral infection, gastroenteritis. If it persists see your pediatrician as babies can become dehydrated very quickly. Signs of dehydration include a sunken soft spot (fontanelle) on a young baby's head, sunken eyes, dry mouth or lips, fewer wet diapers, dark yellow urine, and possible

listlessness. Seek urgent medical help if you think your baby is dehydrated. Never dilute your baby's formula, but you can offer sips of water between feeds. Breast milk has the optimum level of fluids and electrolytes needed to recover from diarrhea, so breastfeed on demand. Keep your baby's diet bland with foods such as banana, dry toast, infant rice cereal, apple, potato, and pasta, until she is well again.

> **"Sometimes babies become constipated when they are first introduced to solids after being exclusively breastfed."**

Is your baby ready for weaning?

Your baby needs to be developmentally ready to start weaning. The US government guidelines recommend that weaning starts at around six months of age and that breast milk is nutritionally adequate for the first six months. By this time, your baby's digestive system and immune system are mature enough to digest solids and she is neurologically capable.

Note that actual age and developmental age are not the same thing. Babies develop at their own pace, which is why the words "around six months" are used. You as a parent are the best judge of when your baby is ready to wean, but never start before 17 weeks as your baby's digestive system isn't mature enough. Consult your GP or health visitor if you are in any doubt.

If your baby is showing signs of being ready after 17 weeks, you could try giving solids. The developmental signs of readiness are:
- Able to sit up with minimal support
- Tongue thrust has disappeared
- Can grab toys and put them into her mouth with good hand control
- Shows an interest in what you are eating.

Remember that sucking is a natural reflex, but swallowing and moving food around the mouth and from the front to the back needs to be learned. If you are doing baby-led weaning (see page 30), your baby needs to have sufficient hand-eye coordination to self-feed.

> **"You as a parent are the best judge of when your baby is ready to start solids, but never start weaning before 17 weeks."**

Getting started

If you start weaning before six months, your baby is likely to still have some critical nutrients (see pages 13–15) stored, so start with simple fruit and vegetable purées to get her used to different tastes and textures. At this stage you can take your time introducing solids—you only need to step up the pace and variety of foods once your baby nears the six-month mark.

If you choose to start weaning closer to or at six months, you don't have the luxury of time. Still start with simple solids, but be mindful that within a week or two you need to start to offer more nutrient-rich foods that include the critical nutrients. Start with one meal a day, then if your baby seems eager to eat more, introduce a second meal and then a third. If she gets frustrated with eating, give her a milk feed first so she's not overly hungry. Be guided by her cues—all babies are different.

Meal planning from six months

Once weaning is established, serve three foods at a time to make up a mini meal containing the critical nutrients:
- Start with an iron-rich protein food such as a scrambled egg or some slow-cooked beef.
- Add a vitamin C-rich fruit or vegetable, such as raspberries or steamed broccoli florets.
- Finish with an energy-dense carbohydrate food, such as a thin strip of buttered toast.

Remember your baby needs iron-rich foods twice a day (see page 13).

If you're doing baby-led weaning (see page 30) or offering a combination of purées and finger food, your baby needs to be able to grasp food. She will use her whole fist to pick it up—the palm grip. At first, more of the food will be played with, squashed, or thrown on the floor, and that's fine; your baby is learning about the sensory characteristics of different foods.

Initially when offered foods she can feed herself, your baby will often just suck them rather than eat them, and this is fine, too. You will find that some foods are swallowed while others are carefully mouthed and spat out. That's okay— your baby is learning which foods she can swallow for the stage she's at. Persevere with these spat-out foods—eventually she'll swallow them when she's developmentally ready.

As weaning progresses

Notice when your baby starts to eat more food, which could be anytime from two to eight weeks after starting weaning—all babies are different.

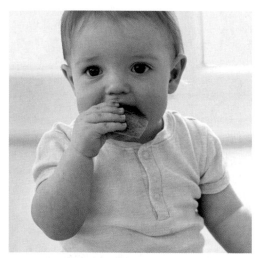

New skills. Self-feeding simple finger foods, such as pieces of fruit, will develop your baby's hand-to-eye co-ordination and encourage independence.

If you're not sure how much your baby is eating, check the contents of her diapers. If the poo is still yellowish, she's still having a predominantly milk-based diet and is playing with her food. If the poo is browner, it's a sure sign she's eating!

Note also her ability to manage her own spoon—this can be pre-loaded by you and self-fed or she can dip the spoon into her own bowl and transfer it to her mouth. If she can do this, that's another milestone reached.

The pincer grip is another developmental milestone, where your baby can pick up and hold food between her thumb and index finger.

When these things happen, consider making mixed family meals instead of three separate items. Try recipes such as Beginner's Beef Casserole (see pages 114–15), Annabel's Tasty Pasta Bolognese (see page 148), and Pesto and Avocado Quesadillas (see page 130).

As a guide, by the time your baby is eight months old, she will be having three meals a day of mixed family foods. By 10 months she should be having three meals a day and 1–2 snacks, if needed. Don't forget throughout this time your baby should still be receiving breast or formula milk on demand in between meal and snack times. Babies have very small stomachs so they need to eat more frequently than adults—they will need to eat something every 2½–3 hours.

Amount of food

There are no recommendations for portion sizes as all babies will eat different amounts. As a rule of thumb, once your baby is having three meals a day you could offer a tablespoon of each part of the meal— for example, meat, vegetables, and pasta—and let her eat the amount she wants. Signs of still being hungry can be an open mouth, reaching for more, sucking fists after finishing, or signing for more. If your baby doesn't seem hungry, avoid encouraging "just one more mouthful" as this can lead to an unhealthy relationship with food.

OFFERING NEW FOODS

Below is a guide to the foods that are appropriate for your baby's growth and development at each stage of weaning—some babies will be ready for a greater variety earlier than others.

Age	Foods	Consistency	Routine
Between 17 weeks and six months	• Fruits and vegetables such as ripe peaches, banana, mango, papaya, pear, melon, avocado, potato, swede, carrots, parsnip, sweet potato, and butternut squash • Baby rice, porridge, cereals • Fats and oils	Thin, smooth purées	Introduce one meal a day initially and increase over the next few weeks so that by six months your baby is being offered three meals a day.
At around six months	As above	Thin, smooth purées	Limit to 1–2 weeks only. Progress from offering a meal a day to offering three meals per day in this 1–2 week period.
From six months	• Meat, poultry, fish, eggs • All fruit and vegetables • All cereal grains • All fats and oils	• Thicker purées or mashed foods • Well-cooked meat • Melt-in-the-mouth or bite-and-dissolve finger foods	Three meals—breakfast, lunch, dinner—with each meal consisting of an iron-rich food, an energy food, a fruit and vegetable. Give breast or formula milk on demand.
From around seven to eight months	• Family foods—avoid salty, sugary foods—and don't give honey until aged 12 months • Give meals rather than separate food items. See planner, page 119 • Small finger foods—e.g. peas and raisins—to practice pincer grip	• Finger food-based meals or chopped/roughly mashed meals • Smaller finger foods	Continue to offer three meals per day. Give breast or formula milk on demand.
From around 10 months	As eight months, plus 1–2 snacks in between meals. Good snacks are banana; yogurt; peanut butter on toast; cheese sticks; boiled eggs; mini sandwiches; breadsticks and hummus; mini savory muffin	As eight months, above	Offer three meals a day and two nutritious snacks between meals. Breakfast; mid-morning snack; lunch; mid-afternoon snack; dinner. Give breast or formula milk on demand.

IS YOUR BABY READY FOR WEANING?

Baby-led weaning

Lots of parents wean their babies by giving spoon-fed purées, but a different approach called baby-led weaning is growing ever more popular. This method forgoes purées and spoon-led feeding. Instead you simply let your baby feed himself. The ethos behind this method is that it gives a baby the chance to explore a variety of foods, tastes, and textures for himself.

In baby-led weaning a range of finger foods are offered to give the baby an element of choice, as well as soft food that the baby can spoon-feed himself. It is normal for babies to play with the food rather than eat it, but this is all part of their development. They will soon progress to sucking, chewing, and swallowing.

What are the benefits?
● It is believed that baby-led weaning helps a baby develop healthy eating habits for life.
● Babies can explore a variety of foods, tastes, and textures for themselves, at their own pace.
● Babies can stop eating when they are full. Although most spoon-fed babies make it clear when they've had enough, parents often persist and some babies, eager to please, accept more.
● Babies learn to manage different food shapes and textures from the start, so they become skilled at handling a wide range of foods. This can help improve hand-eye coordination.
● It can simplify mealtimes as you give your baby foods from your meal and it encourages healthier eating for the whole family.
● Being seated at the table for meals with the rest of the family encourages social skills.

Are there any drawbacks?
● In baby-led weaning, babies can sometimes eat less than those who are spoon-fed so they are at a greater risk of receiving insufficient

critical nutrients (see pages 13–15) that are required in the first 12 months. Insufficient iron, zinc, and vitamins are a concern, particularly for a breastfed baby as formula contains a multivitamin and mineral supplement but breast milk does not. This is where some form of puréeing or mashing of nutrient-rich food becomes important.
● Not all babies are developmentally ready for successful self-feeding, so it may be better to spoon-feed alongside giving soft finger foods. Some babies simply don't cope as well as others with starting solids and need a more gradual transition. For babies who are weaned earlier than six months, purées are a better bridge between milk and solids.

ACCEPTING THE MESS!

While your baby is experimenting with self-feeding, take a deep breath when things get messy. Fully exploring food is an important part of the sensory experience of eating for your baby—constantly cleaning his hands with wipes or spooning food from around his lips can hinder this important part of his development. Placing a mess mat or washable tablecloth under your baby's chair will allow you to recycle food that has been dropped. Invest in some large bibs with sleeves, too.

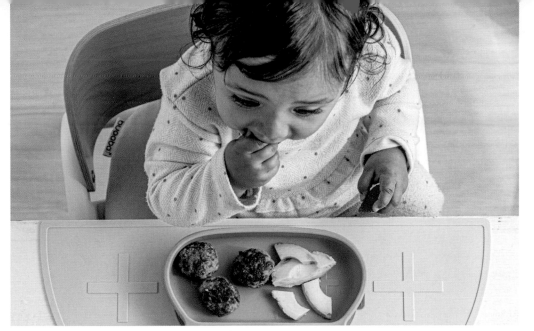

Favorite foods. Due to the element of choice with baby-led weaning, you may get a better sense of which foods your baby really likes.

• A baby who was born prematurely should be assessed for readiness for baby-led weaning. If your baby was premature, seek advice from your pediatrician or a registered dietitian.

Safety guidelines

• Never leave your baby alone while he is eating, and ensure that he is supported in an upright position.

• Be careful about the textures you offer as some will be difficult for your baby to manage. At the start of weaning, finger foods should be soft enough to be squashed between the finger and thumb.

• Avoid finger foods that your baby could break into large chunks, such as raw carrot, and small, round foods, such as cherry tomatoes, grapes, or giant blueberries (always quarter them).

Can I combine spoon-feeding with the principles of baby-led weaning?

Yes. Some parents feel a need to choose one method, but you don't have to. At around six months, you have the freedom to combine an element of baby-led weaning alongside spoon-feeding if you feel that's right for you and your baby. Some babies thrive on purées, others on finger foods, and some on both. Instead of committing to a certain feeding method, it's okay to be flexible and to follow your intuition and your baby's developmental signs.

In speaking to parents, registered dietitians, nutritionists, and healthcare professionals about the various approaches to weaning, combining both methods is a popular option and one that many parents are finding the most realistic to adopt. Offering a mix of puréed foods as well as soft fingers foods at the beginning is also advised by the Centers for Disease Control (CDC). Both baby-led weaning and spoon-feeding allow your baby to explore a variety of different tastes, flavors, and textures.

However you decide to wean your baby, the important thing is to provide a variety of foods (particularly much-loved family foods) and allow your baby to go at his own pace.

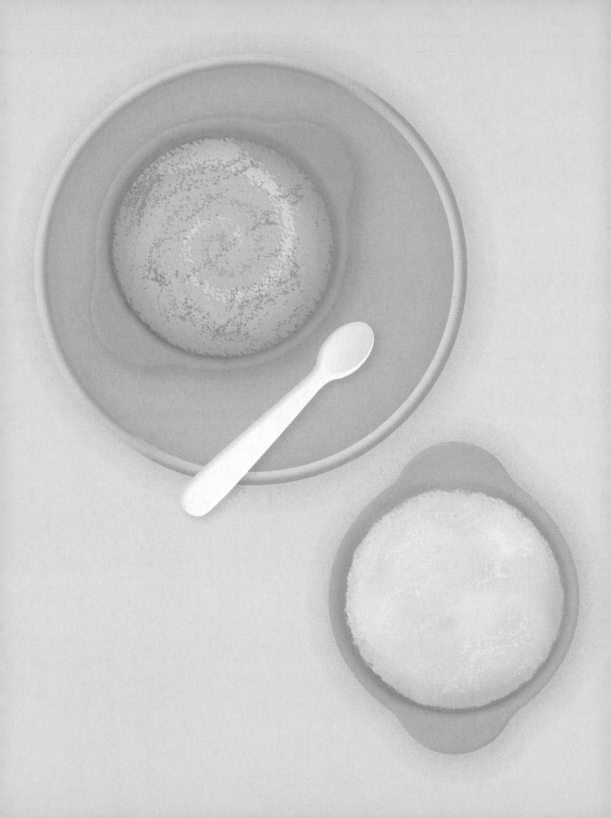

First tastes

Stage One—around 6 months

Your baby's first tastes mark a big milestone in his life and can be exhilarating and nerve-wracking for you. Preparing equipment and ingredients in advance and getting to grips with the best first foods can help make the process easier. The best advice is to take it slowly, spend time planning your baby's meals, and go at his pace. He'll soon get into the swing of things and enjoy experimenting with a variety of different tastes.

• Menu planners pages 64–67

Getting started: what you'll need

A little planning makes weaning your baby that much easier and you'll be surprised how little equipment you need to prepare nutritious, delicious first foods. You may already have most things you need to get started, and buying a few carefully chosen items will help make mealtimes an enjoyable and positive experience for you and your baby.

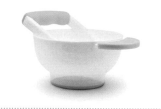

• An electric hand-blender
This is great for making small quantities of baby food and for puréeing family meals for your baby (you can freeze these in small portions and use them as you need them). A hand-blender is essential if you don't have a food processor. Look for a model that has several speeds.

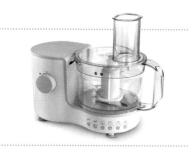

• A food processor
This is ideal for producing larger quantities of purées for freezing, and some also come with mini-bowl attachments for mixing up small quantities when required. Choose a food processor with a variety of blades for creating textured foods later on.

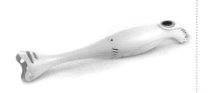

• A masher
A potato-masher, or even a potato ricer (rather like a large garlic press), is perfect for creating lumpier textures. Look for a mini-masher, making it easy to mash and crush small amounts of food.

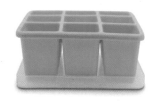

• An ice-cube tray
Freeze small portions of purée in ice-cube trays so that you can use just a portion or two to defrost when required. Choose a flexible tray with a lid. Consider buying several trays in different colors, which can help you identify the contents.

Key

- **Essential**
- **Useful**

• A high chair
Choose one that provides good support, including for your baby's feet. Small babies require a padded insert and a five-point harness is essential. High chairs that can be raised or lowered to allow sitting at the table are also useful.

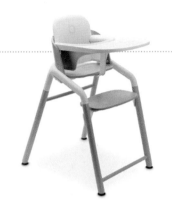

• A thermos
A wide-necked thermos, which will keep food warm or cool for several hours, is ideal for transporting food. This can also be used to carry hot water, which can then be used for warming baby food. Look for a thermos that can be used in the microwave and washed in the dishwasher.

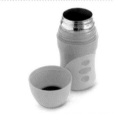

• A bib
Babies are messy, no matter how careful you are. Plastic wipe-clean bibs are useful, as well as those curved up at the base to collect food that doesn't make it to her mouth. Choose a bib that fits comfortably under your baby's chin. Younger babies may prefer soft, cotton ones.

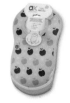

• Feeding spoons
Choose a soft, plastic spoon that won't hurt your baby's gums. It should be small enough to fit easily into her mouth and have a long handle. Special weaning spoons are shallower—they are specifically designed for the developmental stages of weaning.

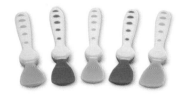

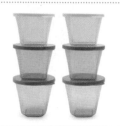

• Small food containers

To begin with you'll need small food containers that you can hold in one hand—these are ideal for freezing, storing, and reheating food, and you can also feed your baby from them (see page 48). Choose ones with lids to make transportation easy, and make sure they are dishwasher-safe.

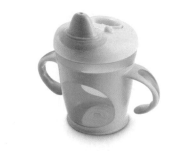

• A lidded cup

From six months, milk and other drinks should be offered in a cup. Avoid the non-spill type as these require your baby to continue sucking rather than learning to drink. The liquid should flow freely, but not too quickly. Some brands have specific flow settings, which can be set according to your baby's age. Cups with soft, easy-to-grip handles are essential.

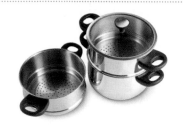

• A steamer

Not only does this provide a quick and easy way to cook fruit, vegetables, fish, and poultry, but steaming also helps preserve essential nutrients, making sure your baby gets the most from what she eats.

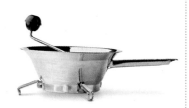

• A mouli (small food grinder)

A mouli is ideal for foods with tougher skins, such as peas or dried fruit, making it easier to separate the less digestible parts. It is also the best way to purée potato as using a food processor makes it go sticky.

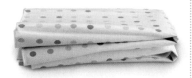

• A mess mat

Placed under your baby's chair, this mat will protect carpets and flooring from inevitable spills. Choose one that is non-slip, stain-resistant, and wipe-clean. Large mats are ideal, as your baby's firing range will undoubtedly increase as she gets older.

Which foods should I choose?

Your baby's food should be as fresh as possible, without any added ingredients, such as colorings, flavorings, salt, or sugar. Choosing fresh or frozen local produce will help you make sure he gets the nutrients he needs.

Fresh or frozen?
While fresh food would appear to be healthier for your baby, the truth is that a good proportion of the produce we eat has been picked well before its prime and has probably then sat in the back of a truck or on a supermarket shelf for some time. If you can get fresh food from a grocery store with a quick turnover or a farmers' market (or, indeed, grow it yourself), fresh is a good choice. However, underestimate the nutritional value of frozen produce. Because it has been flash-frozen, often minutes after picking, it maintains the highest level of nutrients. Some studies show that frozen foods have more nutrients than fresh.

Local and seasonal
Locally grown food spends less time being packaged and transported, and therefore may be more nutrient-dense. Farm stores and farmers' markets are good sources, or you can grow your own. Most locally grown food will also be in season. Fruit and vegetables in season can be less expensive, and are also likely to be fresher and more nutritious.

Raw or cooked?
Raw foods tend to be high in fiber, which is not ideal for little tummies. Raw salads and vegetables in particular contain a high amount of insoluble fiber which can be harder to digest, especially for babies. Cooked fruits and vegetables can be easier to digest and research

shows that we absorb more nutrients from some cooked foods than we would if they were raw. While some nutrients can be lost during the cooking process, others become more accessible to the body. Carrrots and tomatoes are good examples of foods where the nutrition is actually enhanced by cooking.

What's the answer? A few soft, raw, fresh foods (mangoes and bananas are a great choice) make delicious and nutritious purées for babies. However, until weaning is established and they are eating regular meals, the majority of their food should be cooked.

GOING ORGANIC?

Although organic food, which is grown and processed without the use of artificial chemicals and potentially dangerous pesticides, has been proven to be better for the environment, there is little evidence to support claims that it is more nutritious. That said, some parents who make their own purées using organic ingredients believe that they have more natural sweetness and flavor, which helps when introducing babies to food. Be aware, however, that because of strict guidelines governing what can and can't be added to organic products, so read the labels carefully to understand if a product has been fortified with iron and calcium.

Best first foods

A plain purée of a single fruit or root vegetable mixed with your baby's usual milk is the perfect first food. Your baby will be used to the sweet taste of milk, so choose fruit and sweeter varieties of vegetables to start.

It's fine to start with single fruit or vegetable purées. There's no evidence that giving fruits first hinders acceptance of vegetables. In fact, fruit is an integral part of successful weaning.

Baby rice

Mixed with water, breast milk, or formula, baby rice has a sweet, milky taste and is easily digested. It can be blended to almost any consistency, making it an ideal starter food. Choose a brand that is sugar-free and enriched with vitamins and iron and follow the instructions on the package. Avoid gluten-containing cereals, such as wheat, rye, and barley, until your baby is at least six months old.

Millet

This gluten-free cereal is a good starter food for little ones and has a mild, sweet, nutlike flavor. It contains B vitamins, some vitamin E, and is particularly high in iron, which is important for growing babies. Millet blends well with your baby's usual milk and both fruit and vegetables. Simply follow the instructions on the package.

Carrot

The sweet taste of carrots appeals to babies. Cook them until they are soft enough to purée (see page 58). Orange-colored root vegetables are rich in

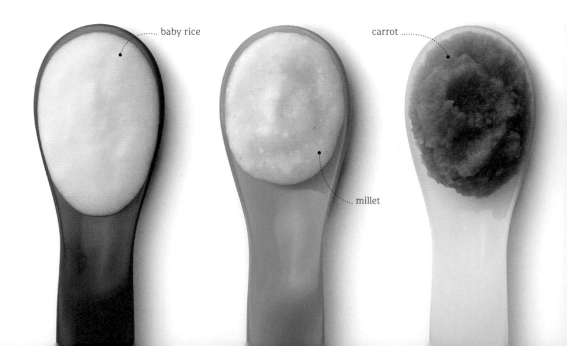

baby rice

millet

carrot

Don't put too much on the spoon.

Colourful food equals plenty of nutrients.

beta-carotene, which is essential for your baby's growth, healthy skin, and good vision.

Potato

Mild-tasting and a good source of vitamin C and potassium, potatoes make a great first food. Peel and chop, then put into a pan, cover with boiling water, and cook for 15 minutes, or until tender. Alternatively, steam until tender. Use a mouli or strainer to purée, as an electric blender breaks down the starches and produces a sticky pulp. You can also bake potato in an oven for 1–1¼ hours, scoop out the flesh and mash with a little of your baby's usual milk.

Sweet potato

Packed with beta-carotene, sweet potato (see page 56) is a good alternative to ordinary potatoes and it is richer in nutrients. What's more, almost any vegetable when combined with sweet potato will taste delicious. Roasted sweet potato wedges also make a great finger food.

Butternut squash

Another colorful vegetable rich in beta-carotene, butternut squash (see page 59) has a smooth, mild flavor. Try combining it with apple and pear, or keep it simple and just mix with a little baby rice.

BEST FIRST FOODS

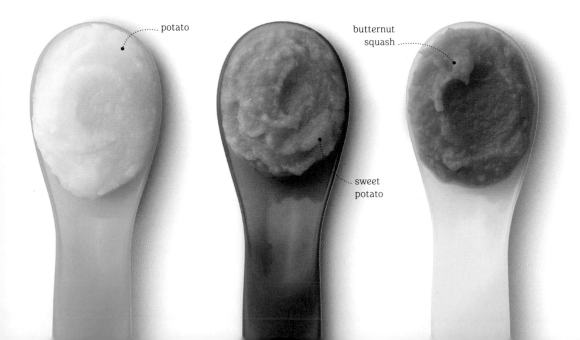

potato

butternut squash

sweet potato

Pumpkin

The orange flesh of this vegetable is sweet and bursting with vitamin C and beta-carotene. Peel and chop, then boil or steam, or bake wedges in the oven (see page 55). Pumpkin purées to a smooth consistency and combines well with fruit, other vegetables, and baby rice, making it a popular early weaning food.

Apple

Apples (see page 60) make an excellent first food for babies that can be puréed to a very smooth consistency. They are a great source of pectin, a soluble fiber that helps your baby's body process solid food more efficiently.

Pear

Pears (see page 60) also contain pectin and have a sweet, gentle taste that babies love. They are rich in vitamin C and vitamin A, and even contain some B vitamins. Pears need to be cooked only lightly before puréeing, to preserve their nutrient content. If the purée is too runny, stir in a little baby rice to thicken it up.

Banana

Sweet, ripe bananas (see page 62) are the perfect convenience food as they can be prepared without cooking, are a perfect finger food, and can also be simply mashed into a soft purée. Add a little baby milk if the purée is too thick. Bananas contain vitamin C and the mineral potassium, which is needed for a baby's muscle function.

What's more, bananas are little packages of energy, providing carbohydrates for growing bodies. Better still, no other fruit contains more digestible carbohydrates than bananas.

WHICH CONSISTENCY?

Your baby's "starter" purées should be semiliquid—almost the same consistency as yogurt. To begin with she'll seem to suck the food off the spoon. The more liquid the purées are at the outset, the easier your baby will find them to eat.

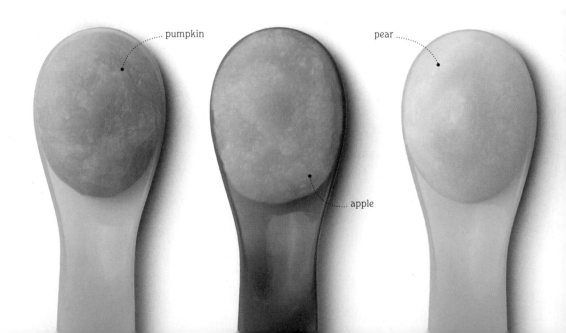

pumpkin

pear

apple

Papaya

Papaya (see page 62) is another fruit that can be puréed without cooking. Its brightly colored flesh is rich in essential vitamin C and beta-carotene, and it also contains plenty of fiber, folic acid, and vitamin E, making it a nutritious first food. Most babies love the flavor, too. Papaya contains a natural chemical called "papain," which helps encourage healthy digestion, and other key nutrients that encourage healthy eyesight.

Mango

Mangoes are rich in vitamins A, B, and C, and contain more calcium than almost any other fruit. They contain a little iron, too. Make sure the mango is ripe, sweet, and not stringy. To prepare the mango, cut it in half either side of the stone, peel away the skin, cut the flesh into cubes, and purée using a hand-blender. Mangoes taste delicious blended with apple, pear, or just about any other fruit to create a wonderful tropical treat for your baby (see page 63).

"Sweet, ripe bananas are the perfect convenience food as they can be prepared without cooking, are a perfect finger food, and can also be simply mashed into a soft purée."

Avocado

Avocado (see page 62) is rich in healthy monounsaturated fats, which provide energy that encourages your baby's growth and development. It also contributes nearly 20 vitamins, minerals, and beneficial plant compounds to her diet.

It's a perfect, nutrient-dense first food and its smooth consistency makes it ideal for babies. There's no need for cooking, just mash it on its own, or blend with your baby's favorite fruit or vegetable purée. Slices of avocado also make good first finger foods for independent babies.

BEST FIRST FOODS

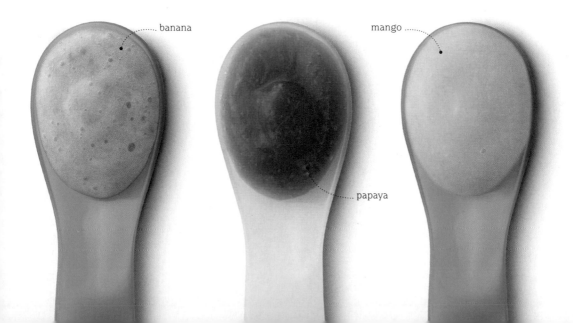

banana

mango

papaya

COMBINED PURÉES

Below are some suggestions for flavors that work well together. Start with the main ingredient and then add one, two, or three ingredients as shown. Experiment to find out what your baby likes best.

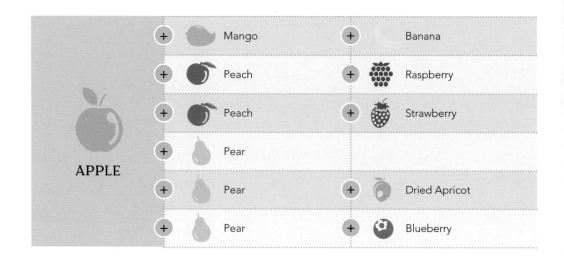

APPLE

+	Mango	+	Banana
+	Peach	+	Raspberry
+	Peach	+	Strawberry
+	Pear		
+	Pear	+	Dried Apricot
+	Pear	+	Blueberry

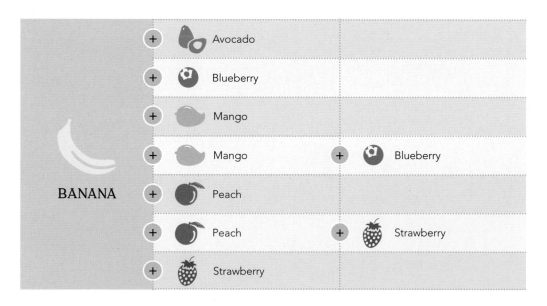

BANANA

+	Avocado		
+	Blueberry		
+	Mango		
+	Mango	+	Blueberry
+	Peach		
+	Peach	+	Strawberry
+	Strawberry		

Combine for varied flavors and colors.

Make a note of your baby's favorites.

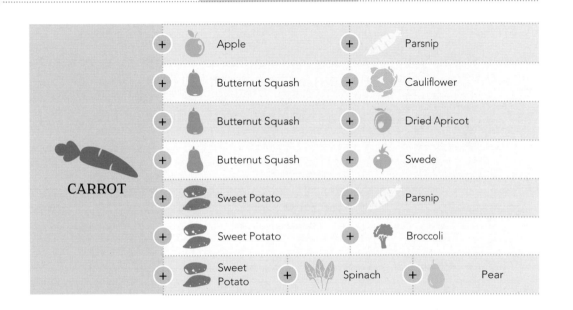

CARROT

+ Apple	+ Parsnip
+ Butternut Squash	+ Cauliflower
+ Butternut Squash	+ Dried Apricot
+ Butternut Squash	+ Swede
+ Sweet Potato	+ Parsnip
+ Sweet Potato	+ Broccoli
+ Sweet Potato	+ Spinach	+ Pear

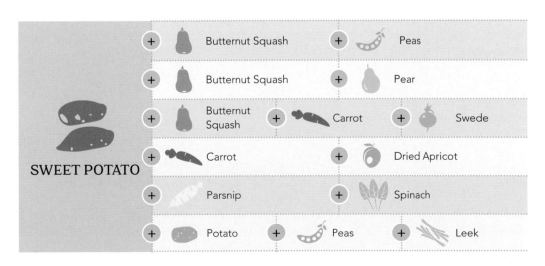

SWEET POTATO

+ Butternut Squash	+ Peas
+ Butternut Squash	+ Pear
+ Butternut Squash	+ Carrot	+ Swede
+ Carrot	+ Dried Apricot
+ Parsnip	+ Spinach
+ Potato	+ Peas	+ Leek

Preparing your baby's meals

Providing your baby with healthy, nutritious meals is much easier than you may think when you first start out. Bearing in mind a few basic tips will make sure that he gets the most from the healthy food.

Healthy cooking
Your baby won't be eating much to begin with, so it's important that his food is as nutritious as it can be. Choose produce that is fresh and make sure that your cooking method preserves the nutrients.

Steaming: This is a great way to preserve taste and nutrients, in particular vitamins B and C. You can place the food in a steam basket, strainer, or colander over boiling water and steam until tender. Or, you can steam it in the microwave.

> "Your baby won't be eating much at the outset of the weaning process, so it's important that his food is as nutritious as it can be."

Microwaves: Studies have shown that steaming food in the microwave is safe and leaves nutrients relatively intact. It is just as good as steaming over boiling water and it's also possible to cook small quantities.

Place the fruit or vegetable in a dish (or microwave steamer), cover (leaving a vent for steam), and cook on full power until tender. Use your baby's usual milk to achieve the right consistency.

Boiling: Although this does tend to rob many fruits and vegetables of their nutrient value, some foods simply don't become soft enough for puréeing using steam. Be sure to use only a small amount of water and save the cooking liquid to thin the puréed food to eating consistency.

Baking or roasting: If you are using your oven to cook a family meal, include some vegetables for your baby. Potato, butternut squash, sweet potato, and pumpkin bake to a nice consistency. Prick the vegetables with a fork and bake until tender, then scoop out the contents and purée.

Food hygiene
Keeping your kitchen clean and using different chopping boards and knives for meat and fruit/vegetables is a good way to prevent food-borne illnesses. Puréed food spoils more easily than other food, so it must be either used immediately once prepared or placed in the refrigerator once cool, where it will stay fresh for two or three days. Purées can be frozen for future use, and will last for several months in the freezer. By the time your baby reaches weaning age, he'll be putting things into his mouth, so there is no need to sterilize spoons or containers, although they should be washed in hot, soapy water or in the dishwasher, at a temperature high enough to kill germs. It is important, however, to continue to sterilize bottles, particularly the teats. Warm milk is a perfect breeding ground for bacteria.

Puréeing your baby's food

Once your fruit and vegetables are cooked until really tender, you can purée them in a liquidizer or food processor, or with a hand-blender. Potato should be puréed in a mouli (see page 36), or pressed through a strainer. First foods need to be semiliquid and similar to yogurt in consistency. Add a little of your baby's usual milk in preference to the cooking liquid from the pan or steamer so that you don't dilute the nutrient value.

Batch cooking

This involves cooking larger quantities that can be divided into portions in small pots or ice-cube trays, then frozen in batches. Get into the habit of adding extra portions of fruit and vegetables to the pot when you cook family meals. Bake an extra potato or two, or steam extra broccoli florets, for example. These can be puréed or mashed and then frozen. You can make up combinations by freezing two individual flavors, such as apple and pear, and then defrosting them and mixing them together.

Freezing and reheating

Freezing batches of baby food means you always have something fresh and nutritious on hand to feed your baby. Once you've cooked fruit and vegetables until tender, purée them and then cover. Allow to cool before freezing. Fill the ice-cube trays or pots almost to the top with the purée and store in a freezer that will freeze at −18°C (0°F) or below within 24 hours. To thaw, take the food out of the freezer several hours before a meal and then reheat until piping hot. Allow to cool before serving. It's important to cook food thoroughly. If you use a microwave, stir carefully and watch out for "hot spots." Do not refreeze meals that have previously been frozen and defrosted. The exception to this is raw frozen food, such as frozen peas, which can be cooked and then refrozen.

KATE ASKS . . .

I find it easier to buy pouches of organic purées, as I don't have much time for cooking. Is there any real benefit to making baby food at home?

There is nothing wrong with relying on the occasional squeezy pouch of baby food to get you through a busy time, but using them all the time isn't recommended (see page 75). Also be aware that the nutritional content of prepackaged baby food could be altered duc to pasteurization needed for food safety for packaged products. They also tend to lack the natural sweetness and flavors of fresh foods, and giving mainly prepared baby foods rather than fresh can make it more difficult for your baby to make the transistion to family meals. Although organic baby food is prepared without the use of artificial ingredients, current legislation governing regular baby foods has made it almost impossible for them to contain any pesticides, so organic is unlikely to be superior in any major way.

Batch cooking, puréeing extra portions from family meals, and swapping trays of purées with friends can helpoffer a wide range of homemade baby foods.

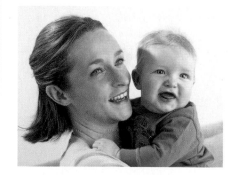

Your baby's first "meal"

Your baby's first taste of "real" food is a momentous occasion and you'll want to set the scene and choose just the right moment to make it a success. Don't be surprised if things don't go according to your plan. Some babies eagerly embrace those first mouthfuls, while others are a little shocked.

Type of weaning

There are three ways of weaning your baby: spoon-feeding, baby-led weaning, and the combined approach (see page 30). In baby-led weaning, you let your baby feed herself. Instead of giving her purées, you offer a range of soft finger foods (see pages 78–79) and cooked soft, but not mushy, vegetables.

Where?

It's a good idea to choose a spot where you'll be regularly feeding your baby, so that she begins to associate it with mealtimes. The kitchen is probably best, as she's bound to make a considerable mess for the first few months—or even years!

In what?

One of the signs of being ready for weaning is being able to sit upright, with or without support. This makes a high chair ideal. As your baby becomes accomplished, you can place food on the tray for her. You may want to use a splash mat to catch any spills. If you choose to wean before six months and your baby cannot sit upright, use her car seat to ensure her whole body is supported.

When?

About an hour after your baby's normal milk feed, and after she's had her nap, is a good time to start her on her first tastes in the weaning process. She won't be irritable with hunger, but she may feel a little peckish. Somewhere around midday is ideal. She'll most likely be alert and happy and ready for a new experience. If she's unwell or out of sorts, leave it for another day.

Who should feed your baby?

If you are doing baby-led weaning, your baby will feed herself, with close supervision from you. If you're giving purées, the first spoonfuls are a bit of a momentous event, so mom and dad may want to be on hand to witness her foray into the world of food. However, anyone can successfully feed a young baby, as long as they are patient and allow her to go at her own pace. Some babies respond better to having dad offer the first spoonfuls. If your baby can smell mom's milk, she might resist her new menu in favor of the comfort of something familiar. Similarly, bottle-fed babies may be upset that they are not being offered their usual, warm treat with mom.

Which food?

Baby-led weaning gives babies the opportunity to explore a variety of tastes and textures from the beginning and learn to pick food up and bring it to their mouth. At this first stage, offer a range of finger foods. Eventually, once her hand-eye coordination is sufficiently developed, your baby will be able to feed herself with a spoon.

The first feed

1 When your baby is happy and settled in her high chair, scoop up a little bit of purée on the end of her spoon and gently hold it to her lips.

2 If your baby opens her mouth, slide the spoon into it and hold it there for a few moments, so she becomes accustomed to the new taste.

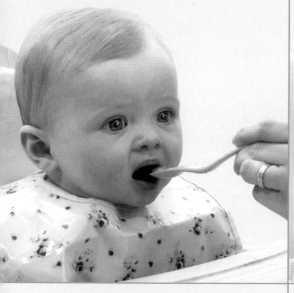

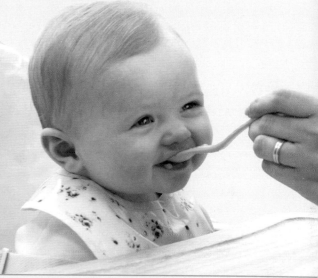

3 Carefully withdraw the spoon, using her lips and gums to remove the purée. She may suck at the spoon or even bite down on it with her gums.

4 Refill her spoon and offer a little more. Don't be surprised if most of the purée reemerges! Simply scoop it back up and try again.

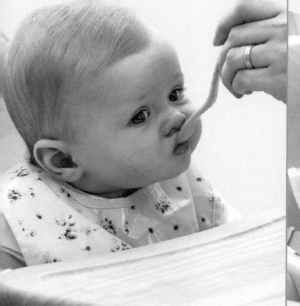

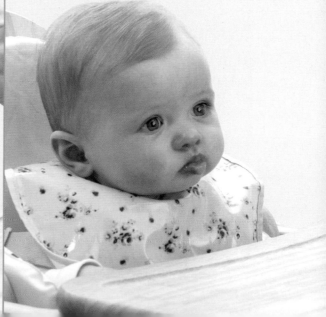

If you're weaning from around six months, a combined fruit or vegetable purée (see pages 42–43) mixed with a little of your baby's usual milk is perfect.

If you are breastfeeding, use a little expressed milk; if you are bottlefeeding, formula is fine. She will be used to the sweet taste of milk and may be put off by the sight and taste of anything new.

Choosing sweet vegetables, or a little baby rice with milk, makes the experience less overwhelming. It's fine to start with single-fruit purées—there's no evidence that this hinders acceptance of vegetables (see page 38).

What consistency?

Adding a little of your baby's usual milk to the purée will make it seem more "familiar" as well as making sure that it is smooth and yogurt-like. To begin with, your baby will "suck" the food from the spoon rather than use her lips to remove it. Until she masters the art of moving the food around her mouth with her tongue, it will need to be liquid enough for her to swallow straight down.

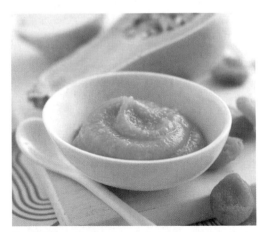

Ready to go. Prepare your baby's first purées so that they have a smooth, yogurt-like consistency, then begin by offering just a few teaspoons per "meal," being careful not to overload the spoon.

How much?

First foods are simply tastes and textures and her usual milk will remain her major source of nutrition. One or two tablespoons of purée or finger foods once a day is about right for the first week or so, but she may want more or less.

What temperature?

Heat your baby's purée in the microwave or in a small saucepan on the stovetop. Stir it carefully to make sure that it is evenly heated through, particularly if you are using the microwave, which can create "hot spots." Body temperature is just about right. Test a little on the inside of your wrist, just as you would with formula, and if you can't feel it, that means it is the perfect temperature. If it's too hot, set it to one side for a few minutes.

Which spoon?

Choose a narrow-headed, shallow spoon that fits easily into your baby's mouth. She may not open her mouth for those first few tastes, so your spoon will need to be small enough to slip in. A soft plastic, silicone, or rubber-tipped spoon, known as a "weaning spoon," and suitable from four months onward, will be friendlier than a cold metal one. Choose a spoon with a shallow "bowl," so that she can easily suck off the contents. You can also give her a chunky plastic spoon to encourage her to feed herself, although she may not be able to do this properly for a while.

Which bowl?

Choose a pot or bowl that you can grip easily, as your baby may reach out and try to grab it. A small bowl makes it easier to scoop up the contents and helps keep them warm. If your baby is very interested in the bowl and spoon, you can try giving her separate ones to play with and explore. This will help make it a fun and positive experience for your baby.

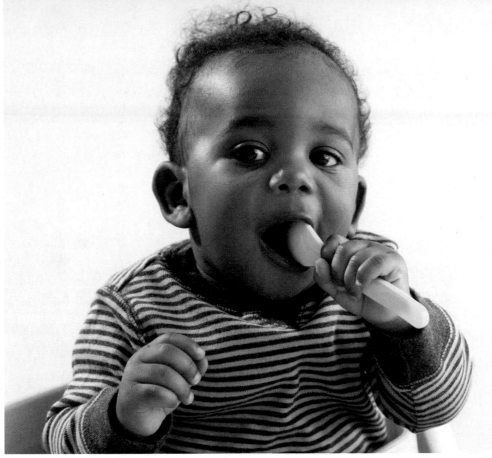

Going it alone. It's a great idea to give your baby his own spoon so he can try to feed himself—or at least chew on it. This helps development of the gag reflex.

How long should it take?

Give your baby plenty of time to get used to things in the early days. She may simply not understand what's required of her, and it may take some time for her to get to grips with the idea that there is food on the spoon. Equally, however, don't continue if she becomes bored or distressed (allow no more than 30 minutes per mealtime). Mealtimes should be fun and pleasurable, so the minute things become tense it's time to stop.

What if she doesn't like it?

Some babies can take several sittings before they get used to the idea of having solids so you may need to persevere. It may not be the purée your baby dislikes—it may simply be the whole experience of weaning. Don't forget that it is a whole new skill that needs to be learned.

If your baby expresses dislike for a particular purée, take it away and try it again in a few days. You may have to offer your baby the same purée several times before she begins to think of it as being "familiar."

The next few weeks

Once you've fed your baby a few teaspoons of purée, or he's eaten some finger foods if you're doing baby-led weaning, you'll feel more confident about introducing new foods. But take it slowly. First foods are all about becoming familiar with new tastes and textures, and the whole concept of swallowing, so your baby won't be ready for full meals for some time yet.

Introducing new foods

If your baby seemed to like a food, make a note of it and continue to offer it. If he doesn't seem to like something, don't give it up—simply reintroduce it a couple of days later, or blend it with a little of his usual milk and try again.

Once first tastes of single fruits and vegetables have been introduced in the first week, you can start to combine two or more different foods—there is a wide range of combined purées you can make (see pages 42–43). However, a diet of solely fruit and vegetables won't provide a baby of this age with important critical nutrients (see pages 13–15), so you need to provide a balanced diet when you are weaning from six months (see pages 66–67).

You will want to make sure that he is getting at least a spoonful of fruit and vegetables, a carbohydrate (such as pasta, potato, or baby rice), some protein (in the form of lentils, soy, meat, fish, or dairy produce), and some healthy fats, which are also contained in dairy produce,

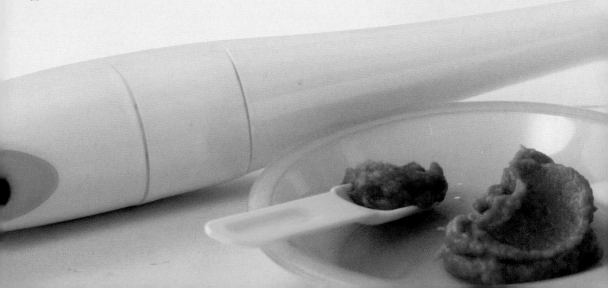

nut butters, ground seeds, and meat. The quantity doesn't matter as much as the variety.

If you or your partner have a history of allergies or your baby has eczema, asthma, or hay fever (see pages 18–24), seek the advice of your doctor.

Combining breast- or bottlefeeding and solid food

Your baby will rely on his usual milk feeds for many months to come, to give him nutrients and comfort. You may want to offer him "meals" halfway through a feed, or at a time when he usually has a smaller feed. His regular morning, midday, evening, and night feeds should continue as usual.

As he progresses toward regular meals, you can slowly reduce the number of milk feeds, or the length of time or amount you feed him. But play it by ear—if he's hungry, he will need to be fed. Until they are a year old, babies need at least 500ml (2 cups) of milk per day. Remember that formula or breast milk added to purées will count toward his overall milk intake. Cow's milk should not be given as a main drink until after the first year, as breast milk or formula is a better source of iron and other nutrients. However, it can be used in cooking or with cereal from six months.

Portion sizes

Don't worry too much about the amount of solid food your baby takes in. As long as he is regularly introduced to a variety of fresh, nutritious new foods, you can consider the beginning of the weaning process to be a success. You may also find that your little one is hungrier some days and eats whatever is offered, while on other days he shows little interest at all. Try to go at his pace and let his interest levels and hunger dictate how much he is fed.

Cooking in advance. Preparing batches of purées and freezing them helps make sure that you always have baby food at hand.

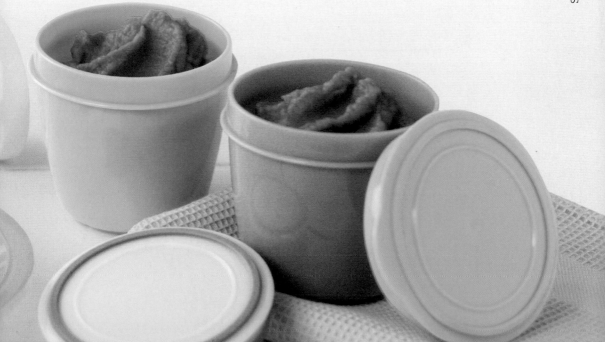

Your baby's response

When a beautifully prepared purée is met with resistance, you may feel that all your careful preparation has gone to waste. There are, however, solutions to almost any problem that crops up. If you're doing baby-led weaning, it may feel as if your baby is eating very little to begin with. The important thing is to avoid panicking and go at your baby's pace.

My baby always wants more

Many parents would consider this to be a good thing, but if you are concerned that your baby is eating more than she should, or putting on excess weight, then you may want to contact her pediatrician. Most babies won't want more than the equivalent of a few tablespoons of purée at the outset, although some are hungrier than others. Make sure your baby is getting enough of her usual milk—she may genuinely need more milk for her growth and development.

My baby refuses to open her mouth

First of all, check that you aren't anxious when you are feeding her. If she senses that her clamped lips are getting a response from you she may well continue—and even consider it a game. Try to use distraction. Get her to look up at something on the ceiling, causing her mouth to fall open. Slip in a little food and

Meeting milk needs. Make sure your baby is getting enough of her usual milk (500ml/2 cups) alongside her first purées.

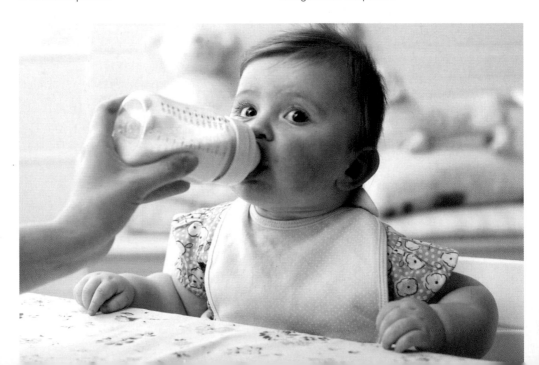

see how she gets on. If she resists the spoon, try either rubbing a little purée on her lips or dip a clean finger in it and allow her to suck it. You can also offer her a little bowl of purée, in which she can dip her fingers (which will eventually end up in her mouth). Eat a little yourself—many babies are happy to mimic mom or dad!

She cries when I sit her down to eat
It might help to have dad or other familiar person feed her. Breastfed babies, in particular, associate mom with the comfort of breast-feeding—they can smell your milk and may become upset when it isn't offered. Try sitting her on your lap and holding her closely when you feed her or perhaps sitting her in her high chair to play with toys. You may need to give weaning a miss for a few days, or distraction sometimes helps. If all else fails, place a little purée on her tray and let her experiment herself.

My baby started on solids, but is now refusing them
It's not unusual for babies to regress—it's a big developmental leap to adjust to eating new and different foods, and to give up the comfort of milk feeds. Try to make the process easier by offering your baby plenty of milk after her "meals." Continue to offer new foods daily, but try to stay relaxed and calm if she rejects them. She'll eventually become accustomed to the new routine, and look forward to mealtimes, particularly if they are fun and you praise her.

My baby doesn't like the spoon
Babies are unable to lick food from a spoon with their tongue so make sure you are using a spoon that is soft-tipped and shallow (see page 48). Give her one of her own to hold, too. Try using a piece of toast to scoop up some purée and let her suck that to help her get used to the idea. There is no harm in letting her try to feed herself, using her hands.

She only likes sweet purées
Babies are programmed to like sweet tastes—breast milk is sweet. It's fine to offer sweet-tasting foods such as fruit and sweet root veggies at first. But it's also important to offer more bitter-tasting vegetables such as broccoli and cauliflower to slowly encourage acceptance of these flavors. You can combine fruit and vegetables or sweet and bitter vegetables to encourage your baby to try these new tastes.

My baby misses the closeness of breastfeeding
Many babies find the transition to solids difficult. Try sitting your baby on your lap and holding her close. To begin, it can help to feed her a little expressed milk on a spoon, to help her adjust. From there, gradually add a little baby rice, or fruit and vegetable purées.

I'm trying baby-led weaning, but without much success so far
Not all babies have sufficient hand-eye coordination for baby-led weaning. It might be better to start with spoon-feeding before moving on to soft finger foods. There is nothing wrong with a combined approach (see page 31).

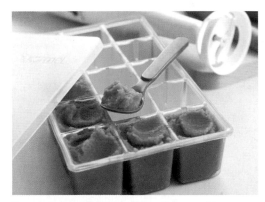

Sweet veggies first. Your baby will be used to the sweet taste of milk, so it's a good idea to start the weaning process with sweet vegetable purées such as carrot.

Carrots are a perfect starter food for your baby, with plenty of nutrients and a sweet taste and smooth texture. You can prepare other root vegetables, such as sweet potato, swede, and parsnip, using this method, too.

FIRST VEGETABLES

Suitable for freezing

Makes 4 portions • Suitable from 20 weeks • Prep time 5 minutes • Cooking time 15–20 minutes • Provides vitamin A, vitamin C, fiber

400g (14oz) carrots, parsnips, or sweet potatoes, peeled and chopped
A little breast milk or formula (optional)

Variation: Place the carrots, parsnips, or sweet potatoes in a saucepan, cover with boiling water, then bring back to a boil. Reduce the heat, cover, and simmer for about 15 minutes before puréeing, as above.

For baby-led weaning, cut a carrot into sticks 6cm (2½in) long and 1cm (½in) wide. Steam until fairly soft. Allow to cool before serving. For parsnips or sweet potatoes, cut into sticks about 6cm (2½in) long. Arrange on a baking sheet lined with foil or wax paper and drizzle with oil. Bake in an oven preheated to 200°C (400°F/gas 6) for about 20 minutes.

1 Put the carrots, parsnips, or sweet potatoes in a steamer set over boiling water. Cover and steam for 15–20 minutes, until the carrots are really tender.

2 Purée the carrots, parsnips, or sweet potatoes until smooth in a food processor or place in a bowl and use a hand-blender, adding a little water from the steamer or some of your baby's usual milk to get the right consistency. First purées should be quite runny.

3 Freeze in individual portions. When needed, thaw overnight in the refrigerator or for 1–2 hours at room temperature, then microwave or reheat in a small pan until piping hot. Alternatively, reheat in a microwave from frozen. Stir and allow to cool before serving.

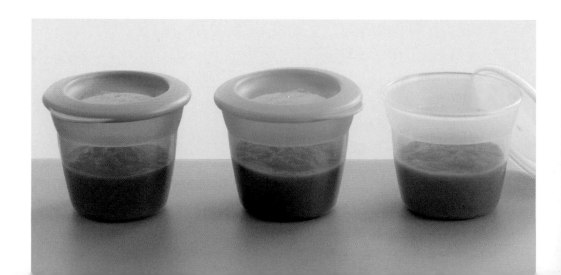

Roasting root vegetables brings out their natural sugars and flavor. Both butternut squash and pumpkin make good first weaning foods, as they are easily digested and unlikely to cause an allergic reaction. Pop some in the oven when you are cooking a meal for the family, and then process until smooth.

ROASTED BUTTERNUT SQUASH OR PUMPKIN

Suitable for freezing
Makes 6–8 portions • Suitable from 20 weeks • Prep time 5 minutes • Cooking time 45 minutes • Provides vitamin A, vitamin C, fiber

1 small butternut squash or ½ small pumpkin (about 700g) (1lb 9oz)
A little breast milk or formula (optional)

Variation: Steam the butternut squash or pumpkin. Cut in half and scrape out the seeds and fibrous strings and discard. Peel and cut into cubes. Place in a steamer and steam for 12–15 minutes, or until tender. Purée until smooth as above.

For baby-led weaning, cut the butternut squash or pumpkin into thin sticks about 6cm (2½in) long, using a crinkle cutter if you have one. Arrange them on a baking tray lined with foil or wax paper and brush with a little oil. Bake in an oven preheated to 200°C (400°F/gas 6) for 15–20 minutes.

1 Preheat the oven to 200°C (400°F/gas 6).

2 Halve the butternut squash. Scoop out the seeds and fibrous strings from both halves. Place the squash or pumpkin cut-side-down on a well-oiled baking tray lined with wax paper and bake for about 45 minutes, or until the squash is tender.

3 Remove from the oven and allow to cool. Scoop out the flesh and purée until smooth using a stick blender. Add a little of your baby's usual milk to thin the consistency if your baby prefers.

4 Freeze in individual portions. When needed, thaw overnight in the refrigerator or for 1–2 hours at room temperature, then microwave or reheat in a small pan until piping hot. Alternatively, reheat in a microwave from frozen. Stir and allow to cool before serving.

Sweet potato is a great source of beta-carotene (this is converted into vitamin A in your baby's body), and a variety of other nutrients. Unlike ordinary potato, it can be easily mashed or puréed without becoming too starchy. It also freezes well.

BAKED SWEET POTATO

Suitable for freezing

Makes 6 portions • Suitable from 20 weeks • Prep time 3 minutes • Cooking time 1 hour • Provides vitamin A, vitamin C, fiber

2 small sweet potatoes (about 500g/1lb 2oz, in total)
A little breast milk or formula (optional)

Variation: Combine baked sweet potato with baked butternut squash for a highly nutritious purée. Lay a large piece of foil on a baking sheet and spread cubes of squash and sweet potato on the foil. For babies under six months, you can brush the sweet potato and butternut squash with a little sunflower oil. For babies aged six months old and over, cut a knob of unsalted butter into pieces and dot over, then sprinkle with water. Cover with a second large piece of foil and scrunch the edges of the two foil pieces together to form a parcel. Bake for about 30 minutes, or until the vegetables are tender. Cool the vegetables slightly then purée in a food processor (including any liquid). You can thin the purée with a little breast milk or formula if your baby prefers.

For baby-led weaning, peel the sweet potatoes, cut into sticks or wedges, and arrange on a baking sheet lined with foil or wax paper. Brush with a little oil and roast for 20–25 minutes in an oven preheated to 200°C (400°F/gas 6).

1 Preheat the oven to 200°C (400°F/gas 6).

2 Scrub the potatoes and prick with a metal skewer or fork. Place on a baking sheet and bake for about 1 hour, or until wrinkled and tender.

3 Remove from the oven, cut the potatoes in half, scoop out the flesh, and purée in a food processor or place in a bowl and use a hand-blender. You can add a little of your baby's usual milk to thin the consistency if your baby prefers.

4 Freeze in individual portions. When needed, thaw overnight in the refrigerator or for 1–2 hours at room temperature, then microwave or reheat in a small pan until piping hot. Alternatively, reheat in a microwave from frozen. Stir and allow to cool before serving.

Any root vegetable will work beautifully in this recipe. They purée to a smooth consistency and have a mild flavor that babies love.

TRIO OF ROOT VEGETABLES

Suitable for freezing

Makes 5 portions • Suitable from 20 weeks • Prep time 10 minutes • Cooking time 20 minutes • Provides vitamin A, vitamin C, fiber

1 large carrot, peeled and diced

1 small sweet potato (about 250g/9oz), peeled and diced

1 small parsnip, peeled and diced

A little breast milk or formula (optional)

Variation: You can boil the vegetables for 18–20 minutes, until tender, before puréeing, but you will lose some of the nutrients. Vitamins B and C are water-soluble, so the best way to preserve them is by steaming or baking.

1 Put the vegetables in a steamer set over boiling water. Cover and steam for 20 minutes until soft.

2 Purée until smooth in a food processor or place in a bowl and use a hand-blender, adding a little water from the steamer or some of your baby's usual milk, if needed, to get the right consistency.

3 Freeze in individual portions. When needed, thaw overnight in the refrigerator or for 1–2 hours at room temperature, then microwave or reheat in a small pan until piping hot. Alternatively, reheat in a microwave from frozen. Stir and allow to cool before serving.

TRIO OF ROOT VEGETABLES

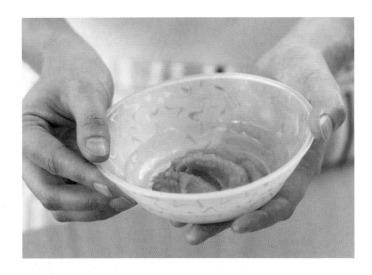

Combining vegetables with fruit is a great way to tempt your baby. All babies seem to love sweet tastes, and breastfed babies, who are used to the naturally sweet flavor of breast milk, will be enchanted!

CARROT, SWEET POTATO, AND APPLE

Suitable for freezing

Makes 4 portions • Suitable from 20 weeks • Prep time 8 minutes • Cooking time 14 minutes • Provides vitamin A, vitamin C, fiber

1 medium carrot, peeled and sliced

1 small sweet potato (about 250g/9oz), peeled and diced

1 sweet eating apple (e.g. Pink Lady or Gala), peeled, cored, and cut into small chunks

A little breast milk or formula (optional)

For baby-led weaning, serve peeled apple wedges and steamed sticks of carrot and sweet potato.

1 Steam the carrot and sweet potato for 8 minutes. Add the apple and steam for another 6 minutes.

2 Purée in a food processor or place in a bowl and use a hand-blender. Thin to the desired consistency with a little water from the bottom of the steamer or a little of your baby's usual milk.

3 Freeze in individual portions. When needed, thaw overnight in the refrigerator or for 1–2 hours at room temperature, then microwave or reheat in a small pan until piping hot. Alternatively, reheat in a microwave from frozen. Stir and allow to cool before serving.

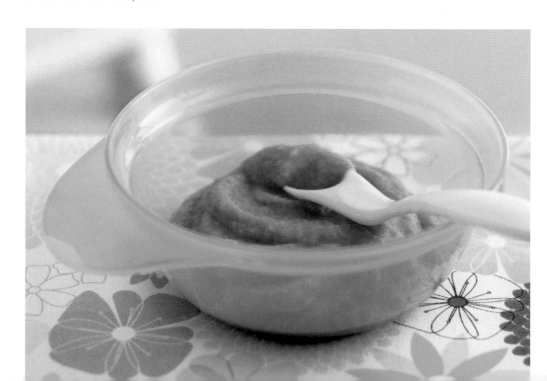

The sweet flavor of butternut squash blends beautifully with the fruitiness of apple to make this the perfect purée for even the fussiest baby.

BUTTERNUT SQUASH AND APPLE

Suitable for freezing

Makes 4 portions • Suitable from 20 weeks • Prep time 10 minutes • Cooking time 12 minutes • Provides vitamin A, vitamin C, fiber

½ small butternut squash, peeled and diced (about 350g/12oz)

1 sweet eating apple (e.g. Pink Lady or Gala), peeled, cored, and cut into chunks

For baby-led weaning, serve peeled apple wedges and steamed squash.

1 Steam the butternut squash for 6 minutes. Add the apple chunks and steam for a further 6 minutes, or until both are tender.

2 Purée the squash and apple in a food processor or place in a bowl and use a hand-blender, adding 2 tablespoons of liquid from the steamer.

3 Freeze in individual portions. When needed, thaw overnight in the refrigerator or for 1–2 hours at room temperature, then microwave or reheat in a small pan until piping hot. Alternatively, reheat in a microwave from frozen. Stir and allow to cool before serving.

The gentle sweetness of pears works well with any vegetable purée. Bursting with nutrients, this is an ideal first combination for your little one.

BUTTERNUT SQUASH AND PEAR

Suitable for freezing

Makes 4 portions • Suitable from 20 weeks • Prep time 10 minutes • Cooking time 12 minutes • Provides vitamin A, vitamin C, fiber

½ small butternut squash, peeled and diced (about 350g/12oz)

1 medium-sized ripe pear, peeled and cut into chunks

For baby-led weaning, serve peeled pear wedges and steamed squash.

1 Steam the butternut squash for 8 minutes. Add the pear and steam for a further 2–4 minutes, depending on how ripe the pear is.

2 Purée in a food processor or place in a bowl and use a hand-blender. You probably won't need to add any liquid, but if you think the purée is too thick add a tablespoon or two of the liquid from the steamer.

3 Freeze in individual portions. When needed, thaw overnight in the refrigerator or for 1–2 hours at room temperature, then microwave or reheat in a small pan until piping hot. Alternatively, reheat in a microwave from frozen. Stir and allow to cool before serving.

Apples are ideal first fruits for weaning as they are easy to digest and unlikely to cause allergies. For extra flavor, simmer the apples with a small cinnamon stick but discard it before puréeing.

APPLE PURÉE

Suitable for freezing
Makes 4 portions • Suitable from 20 weeks • Prep time 5 minutes
• Cooking time 6–8 minutes • Provides vitamin C, fiber

2 sweet eating apples (e.g. Pink Lady, Gala, or Jazz), peeled, cored, and diced
60–75ml (4–5 tbsp) water

Variation: You can also steam the apples for 7–8 minutes until tender, then purée. Add some of the water from the bottom of the steamer or some pure apple juice to thin the purée if your baby prefers.

For baby-led weaning, peel and core the apple and cut into wedges.

1 Put the diced apple into a heavy-based saucepan with the water. Cover and cook over a low heat for 6–8 minutes, until really tender.

2 Purée in a food processor or place in a bowl and use a hand-blender, until smooth. Freeze as described for pear below.

Pears are deliciously sweet and can be easily prepared for even the smallest babies. If the purée is too runny, stir in a little baby rice to help thicken it.

PEAR PURÉE

Suitable for freezing
Makes 4 portions • Suitable from 20 weeks • Prep time 2 minutes • Provides vitamin C, fiber

2 large or 4 small ripe pears

For baby-led weaning, peel a ripe pear and cut into wedges.

1 Peel, core, and cut the pears into pieces.

2 Mash with a fork until smooth, or purée in a hand blender. If very runny, mix with a little iron-fortified baby rice to thicken.

3 Freeze in individual portions. When needed, thaw overnight in the refrigerator or for 1–2 hours at room temperature, then microwave or reheat in a small pan until piping hot. Alternatively, reheat in a microwave from frozen. Stir and allow to cool before serving.

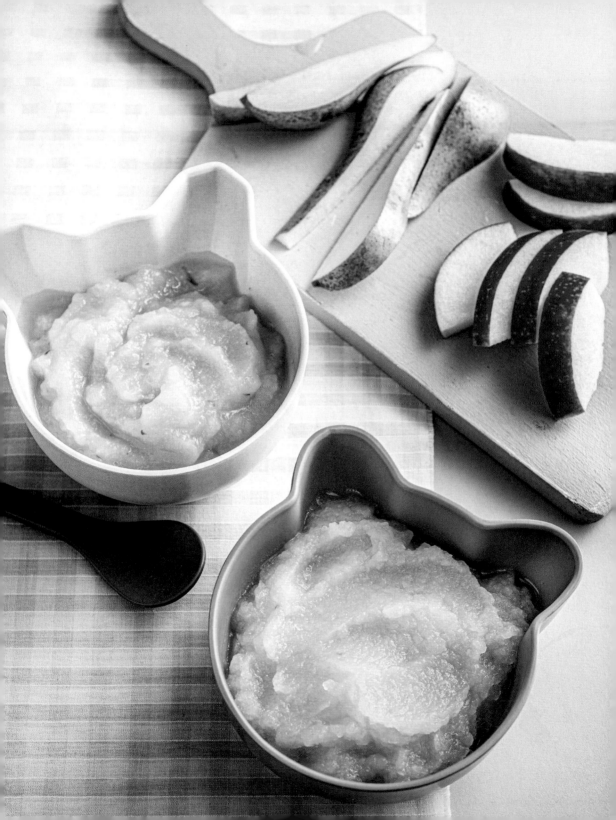

There are many purées that don't need any cooking at all. All these fruits are very nutritious and can be prepared in minutes. They each make one portion and are best eaten fresh, although you can freeze papaya if you like.

NO-COOK PURÉES

Banana

Suitable from 20 weeks • Provides potassium, B vitamins, fiber

½ small, ripe banana
A little breast milk or formula (optional)

Simply mash the banana with a fork until smooth. If the purée is too thick for your baby, you can thin it with a little of your baby's usual milk.

Papaya

Suitable from 20 weeks • Provides vitamin A, vitamin C, fiber

½ small, ripe papaya

Cut a small papaya in half and remove the black seeds. Scoop the flesh into a bowl and mash with a fork until smooth.

Avocado

Suitable from 20 weeks • Provides energy, B vitamins, monounsaturated fatty acids, fiber, vitamin E

½ small, ripe avocado
A little breast milk or formula

Cut the avocado in half and remove the pit. Scoop out the flesh into a bowl and mash together with a little of your baby's usual milk.

Variation: A popular purée combination that is very nutritious is mashed avocado and banana. Place the sliced banana and the avocado flesh into a bowl and mash together.

Peach and Banana

Suitable from 20 weeks • Provides vitamin C, fiber

1 large, ripe peach
1 small, ripe banana, sliced
A little baby rice or full-fat plain yogurt
    or dairy-free alternative

Peel the peach (see tip, page 91) and then cut the flesh from the pit and mash together with the sliced banana using a fork or, if preferred, use a hand-blender. (If you like, you can put the peach and banana into a small saucepan and cook for a minute or two before puréeing.) Serve this purée on its own or mixed with a little baby rice or yogurt.

For baby-led weaning, cut a banana into 5–6cm (2–2¹/₂in) chunks and give to your baby as a finger food, along with unpeeled slices of peach.

When sweet ripe mangoes are in season they make wonderful baby food as they don't need any cooking. They are also rich in beta-carotene and vitamin C. Each recipe makes two portions and takes minutes to prepare. All are suitable for freezing apart from the Mango and Banana purée.

MANGO PURÉES

Mango Purée

Suitable from 20 weeks • Provides vitamin C, fiber

½ medium-sized, ripe mango
A little breast milk or formula (optional)

Remove the skin from the mango half, cut all the flesh off the pit and you should have about 115g (4oz) flesh. Purée in a food processor or put in a bowl and use a hand-blender or mash thoroughly with a fork until smooth. Add some of your baby's usual milk, if needed, to reach the desired consistency.

Mango and Banana

Suitable from 20 weeks • Provides fiber, vitamin C, potassium

½ small, ripe mango
½ small banana

Prepare the mango as for Mango Purée (see left). Slice the banana. Purée together in a food processor or put in a bowl and use a hand-blender or mash thoroughly together with a fork until smooth.

Creamy Mango

Suitable from 20 weeks • Provides calcium, vitamin C, fiber, protein

½ small, ripe mango
2 tbsp full-fat plain yogurt or dairy-free alternative

Prepare the mango as for Mango Purée (see above). Put in a bowl and purée with a hand-blender or mash thoroughly with a fork until smooth, then beat in the yogurt.

For baby-led weaning, peel a ripe mango and cut into wedges.

Mango and Apple

Suitable from 20 weeks • Provides vitamin C, fiber

½ small, ripe mango
2 tbsp apple purée (see page 60)

Prepare the mango as for Mango Purée (see above left) and place in a bowl. Purée the mango flesh together with the apple purée using a hand-blender or simply mash the mango thoroughly with a fork and beat in the apple purée.

The planners on these pages introduce solids to babies who are weaned early (see page 27). Note: a baby must never be weaned before 17 weeks. A young baby will journey through weaning at a slower, gentler pace than an older baby.

BEFORE 6 MONTHS: FIRST TASTES

MENU PLANNER 1

Day	Early Morning	Breakfast	Lunch	Tea	Bedtime
1	Breast/bottle	Breast/bottle	Carrot Purée (p.54) or Baked Sweet Potato (p.56) Breast/bottle	Breast/bottle	Breast/bottle
2	Breast/bottle	Breast/bottle	Roasted Butternut Squash (p.55) Breast/bottle	Breast/bottle	Breast/bottle
3	Breast/bottle	Breast/bottle	Apple Purée (p.60) Breast/bottle	Breast/bottle	Breast/bottle
4	Breast/bottle	Breast/bottle	Potato Purée or Swede Purée (p.39) Breast/bottle	Breast/bottle	Breast/bottle
5	Breast/bottle	Breast/bottle	Pear Purée (p.60) with baby rice Breast/bottle	Breast/bottle	Breast/bottle
6	Breast/bottle	Breast/bottle	Carrot Purée (p.54) or Baked Sweet Potato (p.56) Breast/bottle	Breast/bottle	Breast/bottle
7	Breast/bottle	Breast/bottle	Roasted Butternut Squash (p.55) Breast/bottle	Breast/bottle	Breast/bottle

For baby-led weaning, substitute soft finger foods such as steamed carrot sticks for carrot purée or roasted sweet potato sticks for sweet potato purée.

Let your baby be the guide as to when he moves to two meals a day. Repeat meals on consecutive days if you wish. In addition to the milk feeds shown, your baby may also need one mid-morning, mid-afternoon, and during the night.

WHEN YOUR BABY IS READY FOR MORE

MENU PLANNER 2

Day	Early Morning	Breakfast	Lunch	Tea	Bedtime
1	Breast/bottle	Apple Purée (p.60) Breast/bottle	Baked Sweet Potato (p.56) or Roasted Squash (p.55) Breast/bottle	Breast/bottle	Breast/bottle
2	Breast/bottle	Banana Purée (p.62) Breast/bottle	Trio of Root Vegetables (p.57) Breast/bottle	Breast/bottle	Breast/bottle
3	Breast/bottle	Mango and Banana Purée (p.63) Breast/bottle	Sweet Potato and Broccoli Breast/bottle	Breast/bottle	Breast/bottle
4	Breast/bottle	Pear Purée (p.60) with baby cereal Breast/bottle	Carrot Purée (p.54) Breast/bottle	Breast/bottle	Breast/bottle
5	Breast/bottle	Banana Purée (p.62) or Papaya Purée (p.41) Breast/bottle	Trio of Root Vegetables (p.57) Breast/bottle	Breast/bottle	Breast/bottle
6	Breast/bottle	Apple Purée (p.60) with baby cereal Breast/bottle	Sweet Potato and Broccoli Breast/bottle	Breast/bottle	Breast/bottle
7	Breast/bottle	Peach and Banana Purée (p.62) Breast/bottle	Butternut Squash and Apple (p.59) Breast/bottle	Breast/bottle	Breast/bottle

When weaning from six months, you should progress to highly nutritious foods more quickly to get critical nutrients on board. In addition to the milk feeds shown, your baby may also need a midafternoon and night-time feed.

MENU PLANNER: FROM AROUND 6 MONTHS

WEEK 1

Day	Early Morning	Breakfast	Lunch	Tea	Bedtime
1	Breast/bottle	Breast/bottle	Puréed vegetables	Breast/bottle	Breast/bottle
2	Breast/bottle	Breast/bottle	Puréed fruit	Breast/bottle	Breast/bottle
3	Breast/bottle	Breast/bottle	Avocado, sliced lengthwise	Breast/bottle	Breast/bottle
4	Breast/bottle	Breast/bottle	Sticks of steamed carrot	Breast/bottle	Breast/bottle
5	Breast/bottle	Breast/bottle	Whole Greek plain yogurt	Breast/bottle	Breast/bottle
6	Breast/bottle	Breast/bottle	Lentil Purée with Sweet Potato (p.91)	Breast/bottle	Breast/bottle
7	Breast/bottle	Breast/bottle	Apple Purée and Pear Purée (p.60)	Breast/bottle	Breast/bottle

WEEK 2

Day	Early Morning	Breakfast	Lunch	Tea	Bedtime
1	Breast/bottle	Purple Porridge (p.82)	Lentil Purée with Sweet Potato (p.91) Sliced nectarines	Breast/bottle	Breast/bottle
2	Breast/bottle	Finger of whole wheat toast with butter	Scrambled egg Sliced kiwi fruit	Breast/bottle	Breast/bottle
3	Breast/bottle	Sliced strawberries	Penne pasta with a little melted butter and grated cheese Whole Greek plain yogurt swirled with a nut butter or fruit purée	Breast/bottle	Breast/bottle
4	Breast/bottle	Iron-fortified breakfast cereal e.g. Weetabix	Poached Salmon with Carrots and Peas (p.95) or flaked salmon with steamed carrot sticks Yogurt and fruit purée	Breast/bottle	Breast/bottle
5	Breast/bottle	Finger of toast with cream cheese	Beef Casserole with Sweet Potato (p.113) Banana	Breast/bottle	Breast/bottle
6	Breast/bottle	Iron-fortified cereal e.g. Rice Krispies	Chicken and Parsnip Purée (p.110) Sliced pear	Breast/bottle	Breast/bottle
7	Breast/bottle	Finger of toast with thin spread of peanut butter	Sliced boiled egg Avocado, sliced lengthwise Whole Greek yogurt and fruit purée	Breast/bottle	Breast/bottle

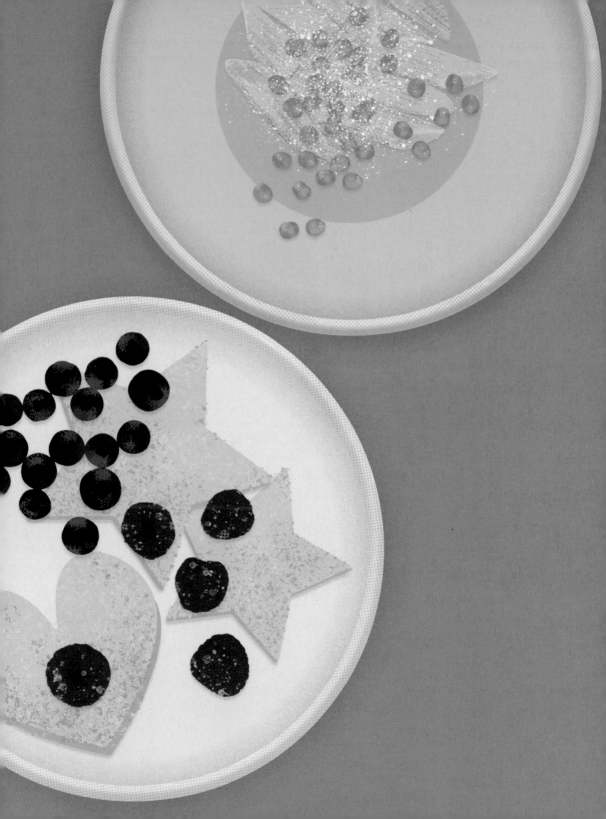

Exploring new tastes and textures

Stage Two—6 to 9 months

By now, your baby should have a good repertoire of foods providing all the critical nutrients she needs to maximize her development. Her diet should include dairy produce, meat, poultry, and fish, as well as an increasing variety of fruits and vegetables. Experimenting with new tastes and textures is a very important part of successful weaning.

• Menu planner page 119

The best new foods

Once first tastes have been established, adding variety to your baby's diet is essential. Choosing from a wide range of nutritious foods will make preparing meals even more enjoyable. You can begin to get to work on creating truly balanced meals for your baby.

Grains and cereals

All cereal grains can be offered from the start of weaning, as long as your baby can manage the texture. There is no need to avoid gluten as previously advised. Breakfast cereals are a good weaning food as most branded cereals are fortified with iron. You don't have to buy special baby cereals which are, in fact, often unfortified and so not as nutritious. Oatmeal and millet contain a natural source of iron and protein. Cream of Wheat and Shredded Wheat have additional iron added, but some instant oats don't, so check the food label. Don't give sugar-coated or chocolate cereals as they are exceptionally unhealthy and are unsuitable for babies. Also avoid bran cereals, because they contain insoluble fiber (see page 26).

Give a mixture of white and whole wheat bread, pasta, and rice to ensure your baby doesn't get too much fiber. White bread is fortified with nutrients, but whole wheat bread has an easier texture for a baby to manage.

Eggs

As a lifelong fan of dipping my toast in egg yolk, it has been fantastic to be able to purchase pasteurized raw eggs in the store. As long as you see the marking and labeling that the eggs have been pasteurized, they will carry a lower risk of contamination with salmonella bacteria. Food safety standards for pregnant women, babies, and young children still maintain that eggs should be fully cooked to reduce risk of food-borne illness. Eggs are incredibly nutritious, packed full of protein, iron, omega-3 fatty acids, selenium, folate, vitamin D, and lots more good stuff. There is emerging evidence to suggest that introducing eggs when weaning may reduce the risk of egg allergy later in childhood.

Red meat

Iron deficiency is the most common nutritional deficiency in young children. In the US, one in seven babies between six months and two years has below the desired level. Red meat provides the best source of iron as well as

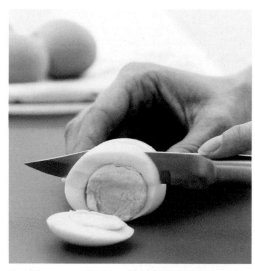

Nutritious eggs. Eggs are ideal for weaning—give them as part of a meal or as a healthy snack.

What's on the menu today?

Get the balance right for your baby.

protein and other nutrients. Babies often reject red meat not because of its taste but because of its lumpy texture. Start with cooked lean beef or liver, purée to a smooth consistency, and combine well with fruit. Slowly cook lean stewing steak in a casserole with root vegetables and fruit, and purée to the desired consistency. You can move on to cooked minced meat, which can be processed in a blender to make it easier to swallow.

Chicken

You can combine chicken with root vegetables, such as carrot or sweet potato, to give it a smooth texture, or add fruit such as apple to give it a slightly sweet taste. The brown meat of the chicken contains more iron and zinc than the breast. Chunks of white meat can also be offered as finger food.

Fish

The importance of fish can't be overemphasized and fish should be introduced at six months. The healthy fats (EFAs) contained in fatty fish such as salmon encourage growth and are essential for your baby's brain development and important for the development of the nervous system and vision. Babies should have two portions of fatty fish a week, but choose fish that are lower in mercury. However, babies can eat an unlimited amount of white fish. Fish is good mixed with vegetables and pieces of cooked fish can be given as finger food.

Dairy products

Babies grow at a rapid rate, so you should give full-fat milk and dairy products. Always choose pasteurized cheeses and avoid blue cheese, Brie, Camembert, and feta until your baby reaches 12 months. Offer fresh yogurt, but watch out for yogurts that contain high levels of sugar and other additives.

> "The importance of fish can't be overemphasized and fish should be introduced at six months"

Fruit and vegetables

Both contain vitamin C, which helps your baby absorb iron, so offer them at every meal. You can purée fruits, add them to cooked dishes, such as combining apple with chicken, or give them as a finger food. Lightly steamed vegetables also make great finger foods.

Pulses

Lima beans, lentils, and other dried peas and beans provide lots of protein, iron, and fiber. Larger beans can be cooked and offered as finger food, and most beans and peas mash up well for purées—push them through a strainer, if necessary, to remove tough skins.

THE BEST NEW FOODS

Foods to avoid

Although your baby will now be able to eat a wide variety of different foods, there are some that will need to wait until a little bit later. It's important to remember that your baby will not be ready for adult food just yet, and you'll need to take care to avoid rich, fatty, spicy, salty, and sugary foods to make sure he stays healthy.

Fatty foods

Babies need plenty of fat in their diet for growth and development and to keep their energy levels high. It is, however, important to choose healthy fats (see pages 13–14) and to avoid very fatty foods. In particular, deep-fried food is a bad idea for most babies, as are foods cooked in a lot of butter or oil, but it is okay to stir-fry or sauté with olive, canola, or sunflower oil.

Honey

Honey is not recommended for babies under the age of one because there is a small risk of contracting botulism. For this reason, infants under 12 months of age should never be fed honey, even if pasteurized.

Unpasteurized dairy products

Dairy products, such as milk, cheese, and yogurt, must be pasteurized to prevent the risk of bacterial infection. Cow's milk as a main drink is not appropriate for babies under 12 months of age, although it can be used with cereal and in cooking from six months and in other forms such as cheese, butter, and yogurt.

Avoid giving your baby soft cheeses such as Brie, or those with "mold" such as blue cheese. Always choose full-fat dairy products, not low-fat ones, as your baby needs energy (see pages 13–15).

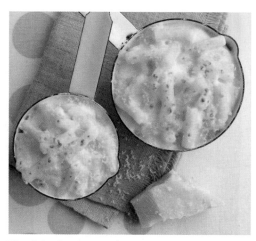

The right cheese. Any cheese you give to your baby must be pasteurized.

Additives and preservatives

Artificial sweeteners, flavors, and other additives and preservatives should be avoided. Because ultra-processed foods can also contain added fat, salt, and sugar, they should never be offered to babies.

Trans fats have now been banned from the US and Canadian food supplies. "Partially hydrogenated" oil was a form of trans fat that was manufactured by adding hydrogen to liquid vegetable oils to make them solid at room temperature. Foods with trans fats have been shown to be highly inflammatory and unhealthy for the heart.

Fresh, whole foods are best for your baby.

Keep salt and sugar off the menu.

Salt

Excessive salt can cause long-term damage to your baby—in particular, to his kidneys. A tiny bit used in cooking is acceptable, but generally avoid adding it to food and avoid buying foods that contain it—processed meats are particularly high in salt. If you use stock cubes in purées, dilute them well and opt for low-salt or unsalted brands. As your baby isn't accustomed to salt he won't miss the taste in the way that you might. He'll grow to enjoy the natural sweet and savory flavors of fresh foods.

Sugar

Babies are born with mature sweet taste buds so they have a natural affinity for sweet foods. If your baby gets used to sugar early on, he'll not only be more likely to develop a sweet tooth but his teeth may also be damaged. What's more, excess sugar in your baby's diet can lead to obesity in later life. Fruits are naturally sweet and root vegetables have a natural sweetness that babies like. Unless you need to use sugar in the occasional baked treat or to sweeten very tart fruit, I would recommend leaving it off the menu.

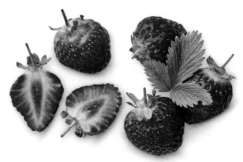

Naturally sweet. Fruit contains natural sugars that will satisfy a baby who has a sweet tooth.

AN UPDATE ON NUTS

At one time, nuts would have appeared in this list of foods to avoid. However, guidelines have changed because there is no clear evidence that eating or not eating peanuts during pregnancy, while breastfeeding, or during early infant life influences the chances of a child developing a nut allergy. Very finely ground nuts, and nut butters, are a healthy addition to your baby's diet, and research indicates that early introduction may help prevent allergies (see page 18), although more research is required. If you have a family history of allergies or eczema, watch your baby carefully. Never give whole nuts to children under five due to the risk of choking.

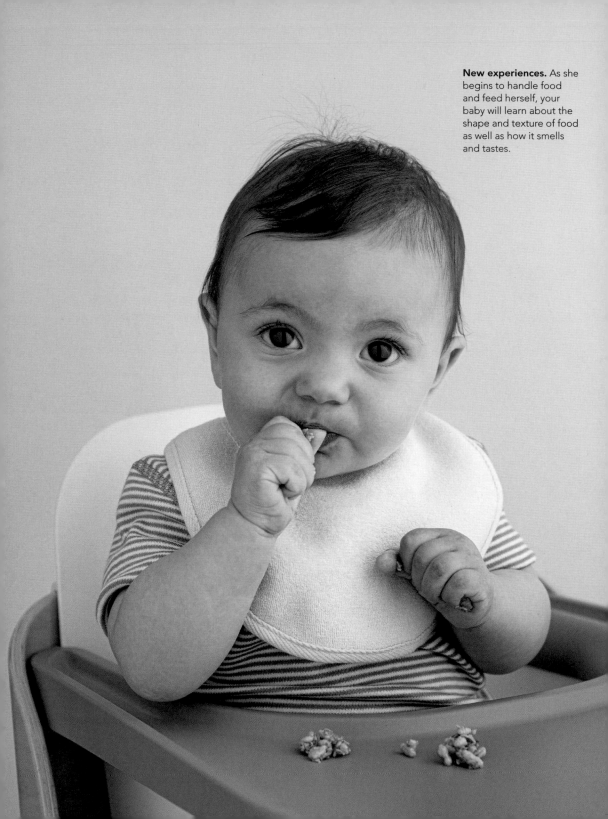

New experiences. As she begins to handle food and feed herself, your baby will learn about the shape and texture of food as well as how it smells and tastes.

Lumps, chunks, and learning to chew

It's normal to worry that your baby might choke if you offer lumpy foods and finger foods, but it's important for her development to add them to her diet—and as soon as you can after she's six months old.

A sensory experience

Learning to eat is a complex experience, involving how the food looks, smells, tastes, and feels, and even how it sounds as it is being eaten. Eating makes your baby more body conscious as she learns to recognize sensations such as hunger and thirst, and learning to chew helps develop the oral motor muscles that help speech development.

Given all this, it is important to introduce different textures and flavors as early as possible when weaning. Even at the purée stage, homemade purées will introduce different textures; store-bought varieties are often of a uniform consistency.

Some parents regularly feed their baby prepared food from pouches and recent research in the US highlighted that therapists are seeing a big problem with babies fed this way. The babies are not being exposed to variations in sight, sound, touch, taste, and smell and because they are sucking from the pouch, they also aren't developing the important motor skills that come from learning to chew.

Introducing lumpy food

Learning to chew is important—recent research found that if there is delay in giving foods a baby needs to chew beyond 10 months, the baby is less likely to be eating family meals at two years of age because she hasn't developed the skills at the optimum time. You don't need

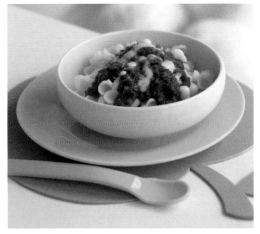

Going lumpy. It's a good idea to start stirring tiny pasta shapes into your baby's purées to encourage her to chew.

to wait until your baby's teeth have come in to introduce lumpy food. Her full set of teeth are hidden under her gums. Some babies are slow to adapt to chewing, but giving smooth purées for too long can affect your baby learning to chew.

Accepting lumpy food can still be a problem if you've taken the baby-led weaning route (see page 30) and not given many purées—your baby may happily chew on soft finger foods, but still refuse lumpy food later on. That's because learning to eat lumps is more complicated as your baby has to deal with more than one texture in her mouth.

Babies tend to prefer an overall lumpy texture rather than a purée with the occasional surprise lumps, so introduce lumps gradually. For example, use your baby's favorite purée as a pasta sauce. You can also add mashed, grated, and finely chopped foods to your baby's diet.

Finger foods

Once your baby has mastered soft finger foods, such as buttered toast, banana, and a stick of avocado, and can bite and chew them, you may find that she is ready for foods such as raw carrots and apple. Keep a close eye on your baby when you give her hard food to chew, in case she bites off a large piece that she can't manage. Always stay with your child and watch her closely when she is eating.

Teething

When your baby is teething, she may lose her appetite, have runnier stools, and be unsettled at night. The following may help soothe her discomfort so that she can eat normally:
- Giving a refrigerated pacifier or teether.
- Giving chilled fruit, such as banana or peach.
- Chewing on chilled hard foods such as carrot and cucumber—you can hold one end while your baby chews on the other.
- Putting a clean wet washcloth in a plastic bag and chilling it in the refrigerator. Your baby will find it soothing to chew on the cloth.
- You can buy teething gels (always choose sugar-free) in the pharmacist. These usually contain a local anesthetic. The gel usually washes away with the baby's saliva, so the effects may not last long.

Gagging and choking

All babies will gag during weaning because their mouths are quite sensitive and the gag reflex is close to the front of their mouths. A gagging baby will cough and sputter, her eyes

"Almost all babies will gag during weaning because their mouths are quite sensitive and the gag reflex is close to the front of their mouths."

will water and she may become upset. If your baby gags on food, it's important to try to let her deal with it—it's a normal safety reflex that pushes food toward the front of the mouth for further chewing or to spit it out.

To help your baby manage her gag reflex, let her self-feed long stick-shaped foods. Once she knows how to deal with gagging, she will have learned how much chewing different foods need.

Choking, however, is when the airway is blocked—a choking baby is likely to be silent and will require urgent assistance.

FIRST AID PROCEDURES

I encourage all new parents to become familiar with first aid procedures for infants and children, either through an in-person or an online course available from the American Red Cross (www.redcross.org).
Note: I highly recommend attending a baby first aid course before you begin weaning.

TO PREVENT CHOKING

Don't give your baby finger foods if she is on her own or if she is seated in an outward-facing highchair.
- Avoid giving raw vegetables or chunks of hard cheese until your baby can chew them properly. You can, however, give grated versions of these foods.
- Don't give whole nuts or fruits with pits.
- Offer large pieces of vegetables and fruit that your baby can hold in her fist.
- Cut grapes, cherry tomatoes, and giant blueberries in quarters.

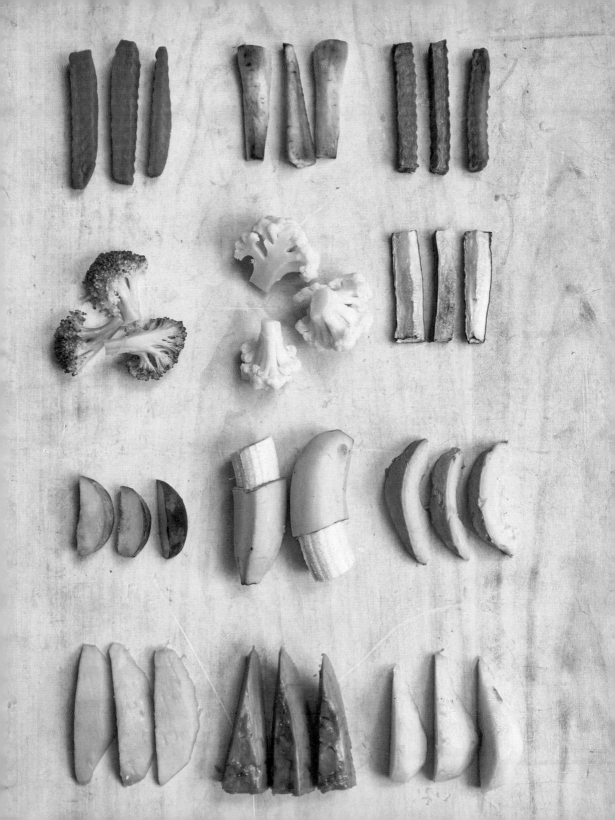

Food for little fingers

Offering finger foods is an ideal way of introducing new textures, tastes, and nutrients, and is also the perfect way to encourage self-feeding.

Begin by introducing foods that melt in your baby's mouth, moving on to foods that require biting when teeth emerge, or when he manages them easily. Good, safe first finger foods are those that can be crushed between your thumb and forefinger.

1 Melt in the mouth
STEAMED-UNTIL-SOFT VEGETABLES AND FRUIT
Offer carrot sticks, mini broccoli florets, and pieces of apple.

VERY RIPE FRUIT
Sometimes fruit is easier to hold when it is left unpeeled. Soft fruits such as pears, peaches, and nectarines are fine unpeeled. Cut a small banana in half and trim the skin back at the base so that the top sticks out unpeeled and the skin works as a handle. Peel avocado, melon, and mango and cut into wedges. Cut grapes in quarters. Leave soft berries such as raspberries and strawberries whole, unless they are large.

MELT-IN-THE-MOUTH BABY SNACKS
There are many melt-in-the-mouth, salt-free baby snacks available to buy, such as corn puffs, baked corn and carrot puffs, and miniature rice cakes. These will soon become firm favorites.

2 Bite and dissolve
POTATOES AND SWEET POTATOES
Small pieces of boiled or steamed potato and sweet potato will be easy for your baby to hold. Sweet potato, especially, is packed with nutrients—bake it with the skin on.

BREADS
Why not offer a little pita bread, a chunk of thin bagel, toast, or raisin bread? Cut the bread into fingers or chunks, but avoid crusty breads that can break off and damage your baby's gums or cause choking. Try sandwiches made with mashed banana, cream cheese, and pure fruit spread.

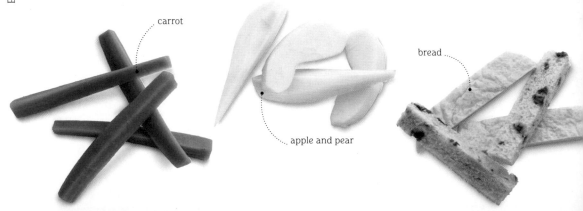

carrot

apple and pear

bread

3 Bite and chew

CUCUMBER STICKS AND LIGHTLY STEAMED VEGETABLES

Cucumber sticks, as well as steamed carrot sticks, are popular with babies because they are easy to hold. Steamed broccoli and cauliflower florets work—leave the stalk on so it can act as a handle. Chilled cucumber sticks help soothe sore gums when teething.

CHEESE

Cheese is a healthy source of fat and an excellent source of protein. Avoid very hard cheeses, which could cause your baby to choke.

DRIED FRUIT

Good choices are apricots, figs, apple rings, and mango. Dried fruit is a great source of iron and vitamin C. It does, however, contain lots of natural sugars. Try to look for unsulfured fruit, which does not use sulfur dioxide in the drying process. Avoid dried berries.

MINI MEATBALLS, CROQUETTES, AND BALLS

Babies love food that they can pick up and fit neatly into their mouths. Try flavorful meatballs and the various croquettes and balls in the recipe section, such as Sweet Potato and Kale Croquettes (see page 86) and Salmon, Squash, and Kale Balls (see page 102).

FRUIT

Once your baby has mastered biting and chewing, you no longer need to steam pieces of fruit. You can now introduce berries too. Berries are "superfoods," which means they contain fantastic levels of nutrients essential for optimum health.

PASTA

Cooked pasta is a great food for your baby to explore. You can buy pasta created from various grains, such as quinoa, wheat, and corn, and these can boost your baby's nutrient intake. If he can't eat gluten, offer rice or buckwheat pasta shapes.

FOOD FOR LITTLE FINGERS

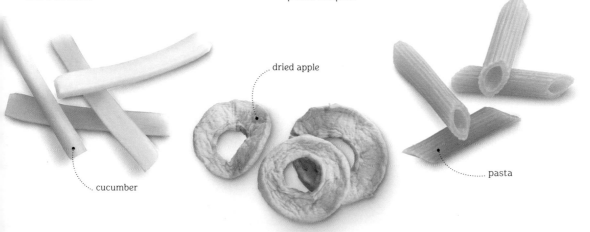

dried apple

cucumber

pasta

Annabel's top 10 weaning tips

Weaning isn't always a straightforward process, as babies have minds of their own—and very distinctive tastes, too! Just when you think you've got it cracked, your baby can suddenly develop eating patterns that leave you anxious and concerned. The good news is that there's a solution for everything. Bear these 10 simple tips in mind and you'll soon have your baby enjoying mealtimes and on course for a lifetime of healthy, happy eating!

1 To avoid your baby becoming a fussy eater, try not to offer her the same purées again and again. Introduce plenty of variety, and if your little one digs in her heels, try mixing new foods with old favorites, until they become familiar.

2 Babies sleep better at night if their tummies are full and they are given foods that keep them satisfied for a longer period of time. It is therefore important for them to have a balanced meal at night that contains protein, which takes longer to digest than carbohydrates. Some protein-rich foods, such as eggs, dairy products, fish, and poultry have the added benefit of being naturally high in tryptophan, which may also help improve sleep.

3 Babies need proportionately more fat in their diet than adults so it's important to introduce food such as meat, chicken, and cheese from six months and not give only fruit and vegetable purées. Cook with healthy oils such as canola and olive oil. Nut butters and sauces made with whole milk dairy products are also good. Don't give low-fat dairy products.

4 If your baby is putting on excessive weight, make sure you aren't pressing her to eat past the point that she wants to. Babies are born with an innate ability to self-regulate food intake and

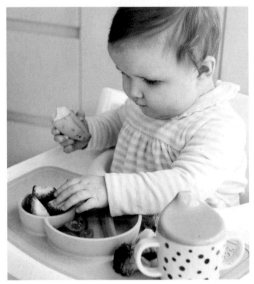

I'm in charge! Don't worry if your baby makes a mess—this is all part of learning to feed herself and also a lot of fun!

no baby needs to clear their bowl. Consider cutting down milk feeds if your baby is getting more than 500ml (2 cups) per day, and speak to your doctor or healthcare provider.

5 Allow your baby to make a mess! Not only will she enjoy eating more, but she'll also be more likely to experiment with different foods, thus developing independent eating habits.

6 If your baby is reluctant to try new foods, hide them in more familiar ones. For example, you can try mixing foods such as spinach or meat with sweet-tasting root vegetables. It's also good to combine savory and sweet foods such as chicken, sweet potato, and apple. Another way to introduce new foods is as finger foods, as your baby will play with them and put them in her mouth out of curiosity. Remember, it can take many attempts before she accepts a new food.

7 Go at your baby's pace. She may enjoy new foods and consistencies one day but turn her nose up the next. She may also be hungrier some days than others. Try to introduce new foods when she's happy and stick to favorites when she's grumpy. If she doesn't take quickly to new textures, lumps, or chunks, don't panic. Try some of the tips suggested in this book, and relax.

8 Make every effort to make mealtimes a positive experience for your baby. If she senses anxiety or disapproval, she'll find the experience daunting and upsetting. Praise her often, laugh, sing, and show delight at her achievements. Join her by eating a little of what she's having and she'll feel part of the family, too, and begin to associate eating with happy times.

9 Never leave your baby alone when she's eating, as she can choke on even the tiniest piece of food (see page 76). Not only that, but keeping your baby company while she's eating will teach her that eating is a sociable experience, and one to be enjoyed.

10 Plan ahead and freeze batches of foods in ice cube trays or small containers so you don't need to cook every day.

WHAT SHOULD MY BABY BE DRINKING?

First and foremost, it's important to remember that your baby's tummy is small and if she fills up on milk or water at mealtimes, she's unlikely to eat very much. It's a good idea to get your baby used to drinking from a cup, so try offering some of her normal milk feeds from a lidded cup (express a little, if you are breastfeeding), and offer water in a spill-proof (sippy) cup between feeds or meals.

Offer your baby water or milk at the end of a meal—these are the only drinks babies need.

Alongside this milk and water, your baby will still need her usual milk feeds, which provide her with the nutrients she needs to grow and develop.

Prolonged bottle use can increase the risk of tooth decay. It is good to start transitioning to a sippy cup with a spout at around six months and then an open cup. You can reserve a bottle for bedtime but it is recommended to wean your baby off the bottle by 12 months.

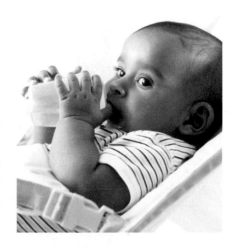

You don't need to buy special baby cereals. Porridge makes an excellent breakfast for your baby and you can sweeten it with fruit purées, such as apple or pear, or stir in a mashed banana, or try this delicious porridge, made with fresh berries. You can use whole cow's milk with cereal and in cooking once your baby is six months old, but continue to use breast or formula as your baby's main milk.

PURPLE PORRIDGE

Not suitable for freezing
Makes 1 portion • Suitable from 20 weeks • Prep time 1 minute • Cooking time 5 minutes • Provides calories, calcium, protein, iron, soluble fiber

20g (¾oz) porridge oats
150ml (5fl oz) whole milk or a suitable dairy-free formula milk for under 12 months or almond milk for over 12 months
30g (1oz) raspberries
30g (1oz) blueberries
½ tsp maple syrup (optional)

1 Measure the oats and milk into a small saucepan. Stir over medium heat until boiling, then lower the heat. Simmer for 2 minutes, until the oats are tender.

2 Add the berries and simmer for another 2 minutes until the fruits have softened. Serve with maple syrup, if using.

To add iron to this recipe, add two stoned and chopped soft dates to the oats and milk in step 1.

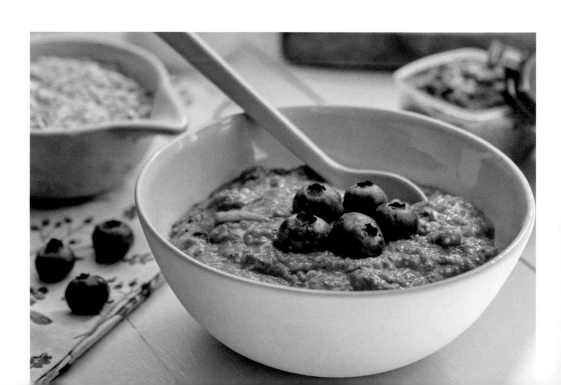

A good way to introduce green vegetables, such as broccoli, is to mix them with sweet-tasting root vegetables.

SWEET POTATO WITH BROCCOLI AND PEAS

Suitable for freezing

Makes 4 portions • Suitable from 6 months • Prep time 5 minutes • Cooking time 14 minutes
• Provides calories, fiber, vitamin C, vitamin A

1 sweet potato (about 450g/1lb), peeled and diced
2 broccoli florets (about 55g/2oz), halved
3 tbsp frozen peas

1 Steam the sweet potato for 6 minutes. Add the broccoli and steam for a further 4 minutes, then add the peas and steam for 4 minutes more.

2 Purée in a food processor or put in a bowl and use a hand-blender, adding enough water from the steamer to make a smooth consistency, or mash with a knob of butter and a splash of milk.

3 Freeze in individual portions. When needed, thaw overnight in the refrigerator or for 1–2 hours at room temperature, then microwave or reheat in a small pan until piping hot. Alternatively, reheat in a microwave from frozen. Stir and allow to cool before serving.

Give your little one their ABC of vitamins with this trio of veggies.

CAULIFLOWER, BUTTERNUT SQUASH, AND SWEET PEPPER

Suitable for freezing

Makes 4 portions • Suitable from 6 months • Prep time 7 minutes • Cooking time 15 minutes
• Provides vitamin A, vitamin B, vitamin C, insoluble fiber

225g (8oz) butternut squash, peeled and cubed
60g (2oz) red pepper, diced
175g (6oz) cauliflower, cut into florets
20g (¾oz) Parmesan cheese or dairy-free alternative, grated

1 Put the squash and red pepper into a steamer and steam for 5 minutes.

2 Add the cauliflower and steam for another 8–10 minutes until the vegetables are tender.

3 Blend until smooth using a stick blender. Stir in the cheese until melted.

4 See recipe above for freezing instructions.

Root vegetables, such as potatoes and carrots, are firm favorites with babies, and the fruitiness of corn makes this purée irresistible.

POTATO, CARROT, AND CORN

Suitable for freezing
Makes 4 portions • Suitable from 6 months • Prep time 10 minutes • Cooking time 18 minutes • Provides fiber, vitamin A, vitamin B1

1 tbsp olive oil
½ small onion, peeled and chopped
1 medium carrot, peeled and sliced
1 large potato, peeled and diced
150ml (5fl oz) unsalted vegetable stock or water
3 tbsp corn, frozen or canned without sugar or salt

For baby-led weaning,
see the recipe opposite.

1 Heat the oil and sauté the onion and carrot gently for 5 minutes, stirring.

2 Add the potato, pour over the stock or water, and bring to a boil. Cover, reduce the heat, and simmer for 10 minutes, or until tender. Add the corn and cook for a further 3 minutes.

3 Purée in a baby food grinder or mouli or place in a bowl and use a hand-blender.

4 Freeze in individual portions. When needed, thaw overnight in the refrigerator or for 1–2 hours at room temperature, then microwave or reheat in a small pan until piping hot. Alternatively, reheat in a microwave from frozen. Stir and allow to cool before serving.

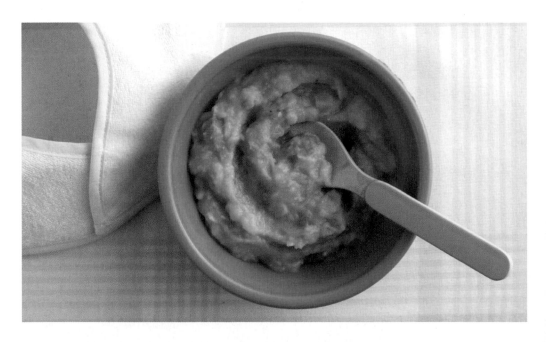

Baking squash in the oven enhances the natural sweetness and adding fresh sage and Parmesan and other sweet vegetables like carrot and corn makes these bite-sized soft veggie balls very appealing to little ones.

SQUASH, CARROT, AND CORN BALLS

Suitable for freezing

Makes 5 portions • Suitable from 7 months • Prep time 7 minutes • Cooking time 30 minutes • Provides B complex vitamins, vitamin A, vitamin C, vitamin K, fiber

500g (1lb 2oz) butternut squash, peeled and cut into cubes
1 small carrot, peeled and grated
50g (1¾oz) canned corn, drained
2 spring onions, chopped
2 tsp freshly chopped sage
40g (1½oz) Parmesan cheese or dairy-free alternative, grated
75g (2½oz) panko breadcrumbs
1 egg, beaten
Plain flour, to coat
1 tbsp olive oil

1 Preheat the oven to 200°C (400°F/gas 6). Put the squash on a baking sheet. Bake for 25 minutes until golden. Leave to cool.

2 Place the cold squash into a food processor with the carrot, corn, spring onions, sage, Parmesan, panko, and egg. Process until the mixture is finely chopped. Shape the mixture into 20 small balls and coat in plain flour.

3 Heat the oil in a frying pan. Add half of the balls and fry for 5–8 minutes until golden. Repeat with the remaining balls.

4 Freeze in a plastic freezer box. When needed, thaw overnight in the refrigerator and reheat in the oven for about 12 minutes.

SQUASH, CARROT, AND CORN BALLS

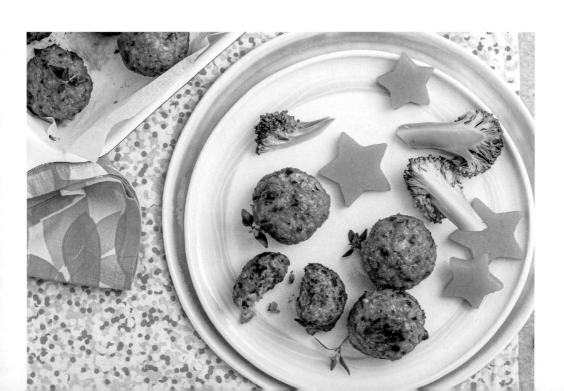

Most babies are open to trying new foods. However, it can be tricky getting them to enjoy eating leafy green vegetables, so that's why I've created these super-tasty veggie croquettes. Kale is such a bona fide superfood that it would be hard to find a reason to keep it off your child's menu.

SWEET POTATO AND KALE CROQUETTES

Suitable for freezing

Makes 14 • Suitable from 26 weeks • Prep time 15 minutes • Cooking time 9–10 minutes (2 batches)
• Provides calories, calcium, protein, vitamin A, vitamin K, several minerals

2 tbsp sunflower oil
1 small onion, chopped
100g (3½oz) mushrooms, chopped
1 medium carrot, grated
20g (¾oz) kale, chopped
1 garlic clove, crushed
150g (5½oz) baking potato, pricked
150g (5½oz) sweet potato, pricked
50g (1¾oz) fresh breadcrumbs or wheat- or gluten-free breadcrumbs
30g (1oz) Cheddar cheese or dairy-free alternative, grated
Plain flour or gluten-free flour, to coat

1 Heat 1 tablespoon of the oil in a frying pan. Add the onion, mushrooms, carrot, kale, and garlic, and fry for 5 minutes over a medium heat. Leave to cool.

2 Cook the potatoes in a microwave for 10 minutes until soft. Leave to cool, then scoop out the potato flesh into a bowl.

3 Add the cooked vegetables, breadcrumbs, and cheese and mix together until blended. Shape into 14 small croquettes and roll in the flour.

4 Heat the remaining 1 tablespoon of oil in a frying pan. Fry the croquettes for 3–4 minutes, until golden on all sides and cooked through. Drain on a paper towel and leave to cool before serving.

5 When needed, thaw overnight in the refrigerator or leave out for a few hours at room temperature. Reheat in an oven preheated to 180°C (350°F/gas 4) for 10–12 minutes.

Flex it...

If you don't have kale, you can use other nutritious greens such as cabbage or Swiss chard.
Replace the mushrooms with red pepper for added beta-carotene.

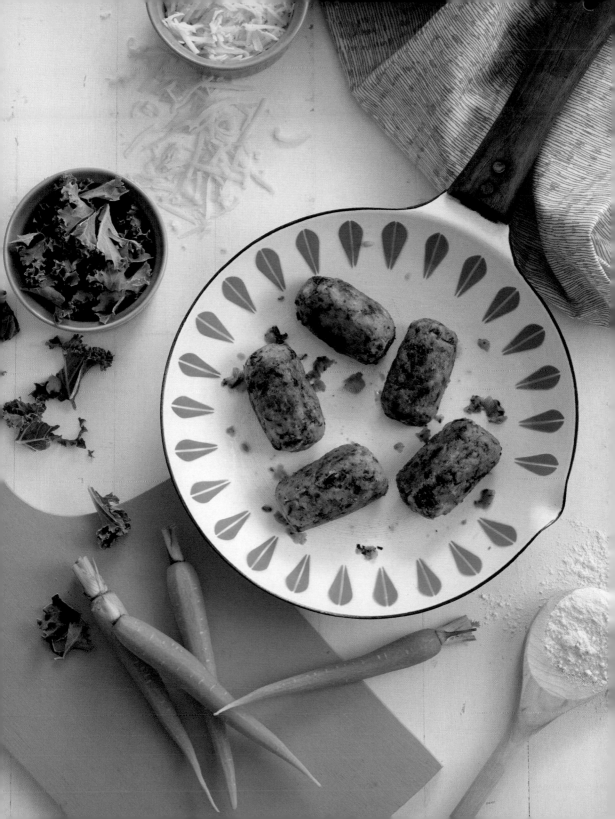

Make a batch of these tasty mini veggie balls packed with superfoods. Unlike some plant protein, tofu is a complete protein as it contains all nine essential amino acids.

SUPERFOOD VEGGIE BALLS

Suitable for freezing

Makes 16 • Suitable from 6 months • Prep time 7 minutes • Cooking time 24 minutes
• Provides vitamin A, vitamin C, vitamin K, calcium, iron, potassium, magnesium, fiber, antioxidants

270g (10oz) sweet potato
100g (3½oz) broccoli florets
4 spring onions, sliced
100g (3½oz) extra firm tofu,
  coarsely grated
25g (1oz) panko breadcrumbs
50g (1¾oz) Parmesan cheese or
  dairy-free alternative, grated
2 tbsp freshly chopped basil
1 egg yolk
Sunflower oil

1 Prick the potato with a fork and cook in the microwave for 8 minutes until cooked. Leave to cool, halve and scoop out the flesh into a bowl.

2 Meanwhile, cook the broccoli in boiling water for 3 minutes until just cooked, then drain. Roughly chop.

3 Put the sweet potato, broccoli, spring onions, tofu, breadcrumbs, cheese, basil, and egg yolk into the bowl. Mix well and shape into 16 balls.

4 Heat a little oil in a frying pan. Add half the balls and fry for 5–8 minutes until golden and cooked through. Repeat with the second batch.

5 Freeze in a plastic freezer box. When needed, thaw overnight in the refrigerator and reheat in the oven for about 12 minutes.

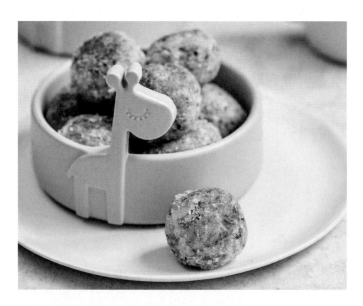

Butternut squash with a tomato and cheese sauce is a great combination and why not save time by using a package of cooked rice?

YUMMY RICE WITH BUTTERNUT SQUASH

Suitable for freezing

Makes 3–4 portions • Suitable from 7 months • Prep time 7 minutes • Cooking time 20 minutes
• Provides calories, vitamin A, vitamin C, calcium, protein, fiber, antioxidants

Knob of butter or dairy-free spread
4 spring onions, chopped
75g (2½oz) butternut squash, peeled and grated
1 garlic clove, peeled and crushed
2 large tomatoes, skinned and chopped
1 tsp tomato purée
200g (7oz) cooked long-grain rice
½ tsp freshly chopped sage
25g (1oz) Parmesan cheese or dairy-free alternative, grated

1 Melt the butter in a saucepan. Add the spring onions and squash and fry for 2 minutes.

2 Add the garlic and fry for 10 seconds. Add the tomatoes, stir, and simmer for 8 minutes until the vegetables are soft.

3 Add the tomato purée, rice, and sage and mix well over the heat. Add the cheese.

4 Freeze in individual portions. When needed, thaw overnight in the refrigerator or leave out for a few hours at room temperature. Reheat in an oven preheated to 180°C (350°F/ gas 4) for about 12 minutes or until heated through.

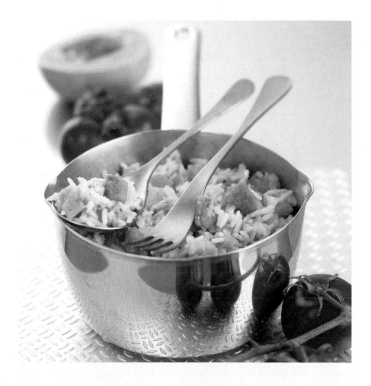

Adding cheese to your baby's purées is an excellent way to ensure a concentrated source of calories that will help fuel rapid growth in your baby's first year. This tasty purée is bursting with fall flavors.

CHEESY LEEK, SWEET POTATO, AND CAULIFLOWER

Suitable for freezing

Makes 4 portions • Suitable from 6 months • Prep time 5 minutes • Cooking time 13 minutes • Provides calories, protein, calcium, vitamin A

10g (¼oz) unsalted butter or dairy-free alternative

5cm (2in) piece of leek, sliced

½ small sweet potato, peeled and diced (about 150g/5½oz)

250ml (8fl oz) boiling water

2 good-sized cauliflower florets, cut into small pieces

30g (1oz) Cheddar cheese or dairy-free alternative, grated

1 Heat the butter in a pan and add the leek. Sauté gently for about 3 minutes until softened.

2 Add the sweet potato, pour over the boiling water, bring back to the boil, and cook for 5 minutes. Add the cauliflower, reduce the heat to moderate, cover, and continue to cook for another 5 minutes.

3 Purée the contents of the pan in a food processor together with the grated cheese.

4 Freeze in individual portions. When needed, thaw overnight in the refrigerator or for 1–2 hours at room temperature, then microwave or reheat in a small pan until piping hot. Alternatively, reheat in a microwave from frozen. Stir and allow to cool before serving.

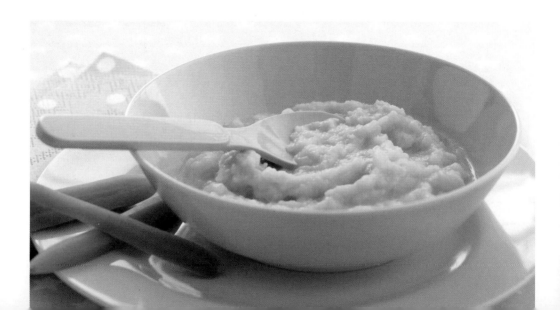

You may be surprised to hear that lentil purées are some of my most popular baby recipes. Lentils are an excellent source of protein and iron, and they also contain fibre. What's more, babies love them!

LENTIL PURÉE WITH SWEET POTATO

Suitable for freezing

Makes 3 portions • Suitable from 6 months • Prep time 10 minutes • Cooking time 30 minutes • Provides calories, protein, soluble fiber, vitamin A, vitamin C

1 tbsp sunflower oil

1 small onion, peeled and chopped

¼ red pepper, cored, deseeded, and chopped

1 medium tomato, skinned (see tip, below), deseeded, and roughly chopped

2 tbsp red lentils

½ small sweet potato, peeled and diced (about 150g/5½oz)

200ml (7fl oz) unsalted vegetable stock or water

Tip: To peel tomatoes, as well as other thick-skinned fruits, cut a shallow cross on the bottom with a small, sharp knife. Place the fruit in a bowl, cover with boiling water, then leave for 30–60 seconds. Drain and rinse in cold water. When the fruit is cool enough to handle, find the cross you made. Grasp a corner of loose skin and gently pull off the skin.

1 Heat the oil in a pan and sauté the onion and red pepper gently, stirring, for 4 minutes until softened. Add the tomato and sauté, stirring, for 1 minute.

2 Rinse the lentils, add them to the pan along with the sweet potato, and pour over the vegetable stock or water. Bring to a boil, reduce the heat, cover, and simmer for 20–25 minutes, or until the lentils are quite mushy. Top up with a little more water if necessary, but there should be only a little liquid left in the pan at the end.

3 Purée until smooth in a food processor or place in a bowl and use a hand-blender.

4 Freeze in individual portions. When needed, thaw overnight in the refrigerator or for 1–2 hours at room temperature, then microwave or reheat in a small pan until piping hot. Alternatively, reheat in a microwave from frozen. Stir and allow to cool before serving.

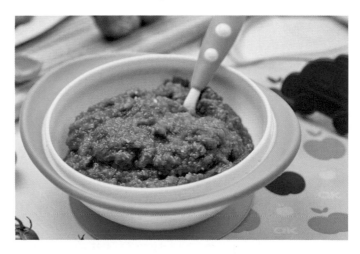

LENTIL PURÉE WITH SWEET POTATO

Rich, sweet, and full of antioxidants and other nutrients, this creamy pasta dish will appeal to babies and children of all ages. You can freeze the sauce separately in individual portions then thaw, reheat, and add to freshly cooked pasta before serving if you prefer.

TOMATO AND BUTTERNUT SQUASH PASTA

Suitable for freezing

Makes 5 portions • Suitable from 6 months • Prep time 10 minutes • Cooking time 40 minutes • Provides calories, protein, vitamin A, fiber

2 tsp light olive oil
½ small red onion, peeled and finely chopped
1 tsp freshly chopped thyme or ¼ tsp dried thyme
125g (4½oz) peeled and diced butternut squash
1 garlic clove, peeled and crushed
400g (14oz) can chopped tomatoes
75ml (5 tbsp) water
½ tsp sun-dried tomato paste or tomato purée
30g (1oz) Cheddar cheese or dairy-free alternative, grated
1 tbsp double cream or dairy-free alternative
75g (2½oz) elbow pasta or wheat- or gluten-free pasta

1 Heat the oil in a saucepan. Add the onion, thyme, and butternut squash. Sauté, stirring, over a low heat for 5 minutes. Add the garlic and cook for a further 1 minute.

2 Add the remaining ingredients except the cheese, cream, and pasta. Bring to the boil, reduce the heat, and simmer gently for 30 minutes, or until soft and pulpy, stirring occasionally.

3 Add the cheese and purée the mixture until smooth in a food processor or place in a bowl and use a hand-blender. Mix in the cream.

4 Meanwhile, cook the pasta in a large saucepan of lightly salted water according to the package instructions. Leave out salt for babies under one. Drain. Stir in the tomato and butternut squash sauce. Serve with grated cheese or a dairy-free alternative, if you wish.

5 Freeze in individual portions. When needed, thaw overnight in the refrigerator or for 1–2 hours at room temperature, then microwave or reheat in a small pan until piping hot. Stir and allow to cool before serving.

Flex it...

Replace the thyme
with the same quantity of dried or fresh basil, which is considered to be one of the healthiest herbs.

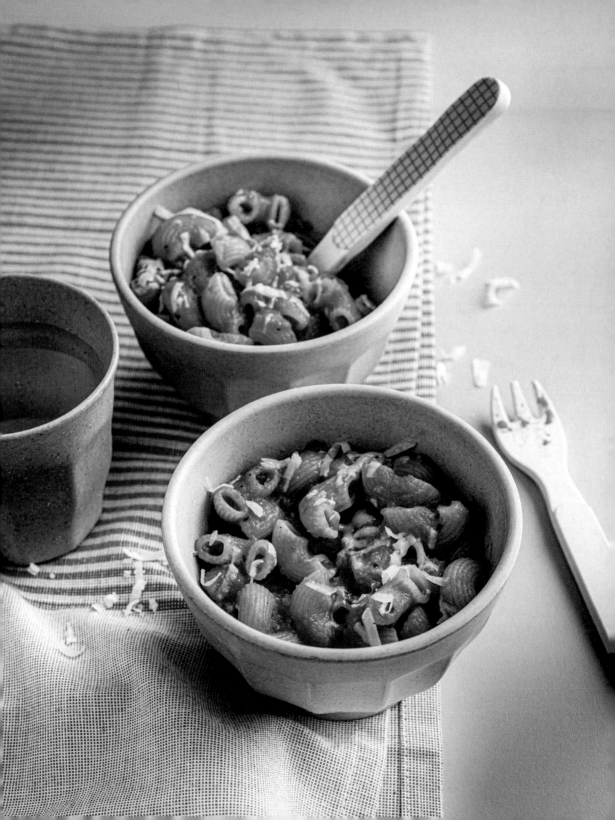

This nourishing chowder makes a perfect meal for a hungry baby. In fact, the whole family will enjoy the rich, delicious flavors.

SALMON AND CORN CHOWDER

Suitable for freezing

Makes 5 portions • Suitable from 6 months • Prep time 10 minutes • Cooking time 22 minutes • Provides calories, protein, omega-3 EFAs, fiber, vitamin D, vitamin B12

1 tbsp olive oil

1 small onion, peeled and chopped

2 medium carrots, peeled and diced

½ stick celery, strings removed (see tip, below) and chopped

1 medium potato, peeled and diced

1 small garlic clove, peeled and crushed

100ml (3½fl oz) unsalted vegetable stock or water

100ml (3½fl oz) whole milk or a suitable dairy-free formula milk for under 12 months or almond milk for over 12 months

115g (4oz) boneless salmon fillet, skinned and cut into small cubes

100g (3½oz) canned corn (with no added sugar or salt) packed in water, drained

Tip: The easiest way to remove strings from celery is to peel the sticks with a potato peeler. This prevents unpleasant strands from appearing in the finished dish.

1 Heat the oil in a saucepan. Stir in the onion, carrots, celery, and potato. Reduce the heat as low as possible, cover, and cook very gently for 10 minutes, stirring occasionally. Add the garlic and stir for 30 seconds.

2 Add the stock or water, bring to the boil, cover, and cook for 8 minutes until tender. Add the milk, salmon, and corn, bring back to the boil, reduce the heat again, and cook gently for a further 4 minutes.

3 Purée until smooth in a food processor or place in a bowl and use a hand-blender. For older babies, mash with a fork.

4 Freeze in individual portions. When needed, thaw overnight in the refrigerator or for 1–2 hours at room temperature, then microwave or reheat in a small pan until piping hot. Alternatively, reheat in a microwave from frozen. Stir and allow to cool before serving.

Flex it...

Replace the carrots
with the same quantity of zuccini, which are packed with immune-boosting vitamin C.

Use a sweet potato—they contain more fiber and vitamin A than a standard white potato.

It's hard to find a jar of baby purée that contains fatty fish such as salmon, yet the essential fatty acids in fatty fish are particularly important for the development of your baby's brain, nervous system, and vision, and ideally should be included in his diet twice a week. Did you know that fats such as these are also one of the principal sources of calories in breast milk?

POACHED SALMON WITH CARROTS AND PEAS

Suitable for freezing

Makes 3 portions • Suitable from 6 months • Prep time 8 minutes • Cooking time 11 minutes
• Provides calories, protein, omega-3 EFAs, fiber, vitamin D, vitamin B12

150ml (5fl oz) unsalted vegetable stock or water

1 small potato, peeled and diced

1 medium carrot, peeled and diced

100g (3½oz) boneless salmon fillet, skinned and cut into small cubes

2 tbsp frozen peas

45g (1½oz) Cheddar cheese or dairy-free alternative, grated

1 Put the stock or water in a saucepan with the potato and carrot. Bring to the boil, then cook over a medium heat for 7–8 minutes, or until the potato and carrot are just tender.

2 Add the salmon and peas. Cover again and simmer for 3 minutes, until the fish flakes easily and the vegetables are tender. Remove from the heat and stir in the grated cheese.

3 Purée until smooth in a food processor or place in a bowl and use a hand-blender. For older babies, mash with a fork.

4 Freeze in individual portions. When needed, thaw overnight in the refrigerator or for 1–2 hours at room temperature, then microwave or reheat in a small pan until piping hot. Alternatively, reheat in a microwave from frozen. Stir and allow to cool before serving.

POACHED SALMON WITH CARROTS AND PEAS

Flex it...

Replace the salmon
with the same quantity of cod or pollock, which is also a source of omega-3 fatty acids.

Use the same quantity of frozen mixed vegetables in place of the peas.

White fish such as cod is an excellent source of high-value protein. The cheese and milk in this dish provide calcium, which is essential to bone health. You can add a little less milk to this recipe if you are making it for an older baby.

COD WITH BUTTERNUT SQUASH AND CHEESE SAUCE

Suitable for freezing
Makes 4 portions • Suitable from 28 weeks • Prep time 10 minutes • Cooking time 11 minutes • Provides calories, calcium, vitamin B12, vitamin A, protein

15g (½oz) unsalted butter or dairy-free spread

½ small onion, peeled and finely chopped

85g (3oz) peeled and diced butternut squash

15g (½oz) plain flour or gluten-free flour

75ml (5 tbsp) whole milk or a suitable dairy-free formula milk for under 12 months or almond milk for over 12 months

75ml (5 tbsp) unsalted vegetable stock or water

100g (3½oz) cod fillet, skinned and cut into small cubes

30g (1oz) Parmesan cheese or dairy-free alternative, grated

1 Melt the butter in a saucepan and stir in the onion and butternut squash. Reduce the heat as low as possible, cover, and cook very gently for 5 minutes until soft, stirring occasionally.

2 Stir in the flour and cook for 1 minute. Remove from the heat, gradually add the milk and stock or water, return to the heat, bring to the boil, and simmer for 2 minutes, stirring.

3 Add the cubes of fish and cook for 2–3 minutes, until tender and cooked through.

4 Add the cheese and purée the mixture until smooth in a food processor or place in a bowl and use a hand-blender. For older babies, mash with a fork.

5 Freeze in individual portions. Thaw overnight in the refrigerator or for 1–2 hours at room temperature, then microwave or reheat in a small pan until piping hot. Stir and allow to cool before serving.

For baby-led weaning, place the cod fillet on a piece of foil with a knob of butter, wrap it up as a parcel, and bake in the oven at 180°C (350°F)/gas 4) for about 15 minutes. Once cooled, your baby can pick up and eat the perfectly cooked pieces of cod. Serve with some steamed vegetables, such as broccoli. See also the recipe on the opposite page.

Flex it...
Replace the cod with plaice or hake, which are equally nutritious.
Use any winter squash in place of the butternut.

If you've chosen the baby-led weaning route, you can take the same ingredients as for the recipe opposite, add some fresh sage and a little sweet chili, and process everything together to make these tasty croquettes.

COD AND SQUASH CROQUETTES

Suitable for freezing

Makes 10 • Suitable from 28 weeks • Prep time 10 minutes • Cooking time 12 minutes
• Provides calories, protein, vitamin A, calcium

½ onion, diced

85g (3oz) peeled and grated butternut squash

100g (3½oz) cod fillet, skinned and cut into small cubes

30g (1oz) Parmesan cheese or dairy-free alternative, grated

70g (2½oz) breadcrumbs or gluten-free breadcrumbs

1 tsp sweet chili sauce

1 tsp freshly chopped sage

Plain flour or gluten-free flour

1 tbsp sunflower oil, for frying

1 Place all the ingredients except the flour and oil in a food processor. Process until finely chopped. Shape into 10 croquette shapes and roll in the flour.

2 Heat the oil in a frying pan. Fry the croquettes for 10–12 minutes over a medium heat, until golden on all sides and cooked through. Drain on kitchen paper and leave to cool before serving.

3 When needed, thaw overnight in the refrigerator or leave out for a few hours at room temperature. Reheat in an oven preheated to 180°C (350°F/gas 4) for 10–12 minutes.

COD AND SQUASH CROQUETTES

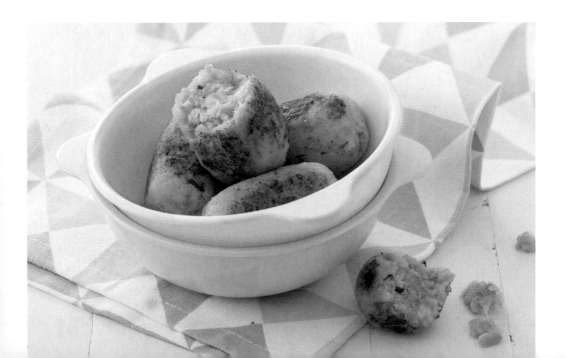

This flavorful fish purée is packed with protein and vitamins, making it the perfect way to make sure your baby gets the nutrients she needs. Miss out the puréeing stage and top with mashed potatoes for a delicious family fish pie.

SPINACH AND COD PURÉE

Suitable for freezing

Makes 3 portions • Suitable from 6 months • Prep time 8 minutes • Cooking time 16 minutes • Provides calories, protein, calcium, vitamin K, vitamin B12

15g (½oz) unsalted butter or dairy-free spread

5cm (2in) piece of leek, finely sliced

1 medium potato, peeled and diced

100ml (3½fl oz) unsalted vegetable stock or water

75ml (5 tbsp) whole milk or a suitable dairy-free formula milk for under 12 months or almond milk for over 12 months

2 handfuls baby spinach leaves, roughly chopped

100g (3½oz) boneless cod fillet or other white fish, skinned and cut into small cubes

15g (½oz) Parmesan cheese or dairy-free alternative, grated

1 Heat the butter in a saucepan. Add the leek and sauté gently, stirring, for 3 minutes. Add the potato and sauté, stirring, for 2 minutes.

2 Add the stock or water and milk. Bring to a boil, reduce the heat, cover, and simmer for 8 minutes, until the vegetables are tender.

3 Add the spinach and cod and stir over the heat for 3 minutes, or until the spinach has wilted and the cod is cooked. Stir in the cheese and purée until smooth in a food processor or place in a bowl and use a hand-blender. For older babies, mash with a fork.

4 Freeze in individual portions. When needed, thaw overnight in the refrigerator or for 1–2 hours at room temperature, then microwave or reheat in a small pan until piping hot. Alternatively, microwave from frozen. Stir and allow to cool before serving.

Flex it...

Use Swiss chard instead of spinach. This nutrient-rich vegetable is a great source of vitamins K, A, and C.

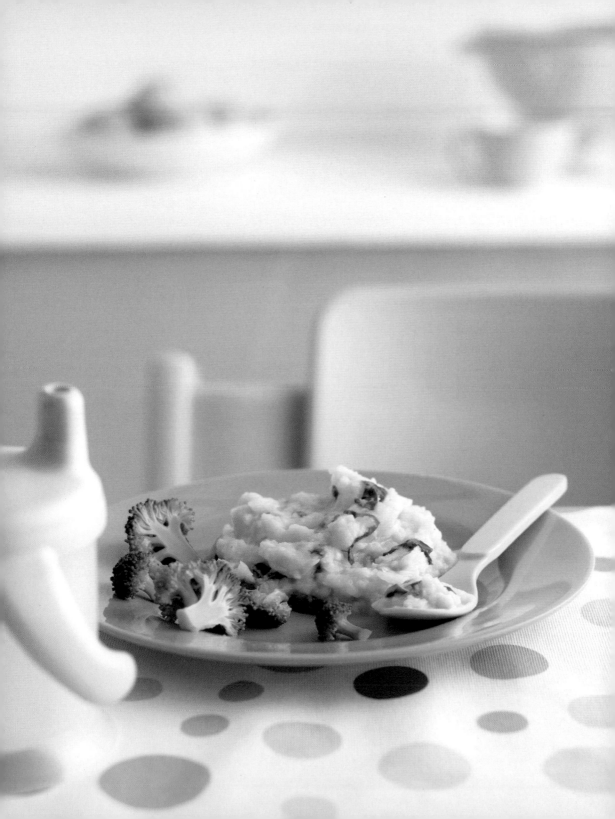

It's never too early to establish fatty fish on the menu, and this salmon purée provides lots of EFAs to encourage healthy growth and development.

ANNABEL'S TASTY SALMON

Suitable for freezing
Makes 2 portions • Suitable from 6 months • Prep time 5 minutes • Cooking time 15 minutes • Provides protein, omega-3 EFAs, vitamin D, vitamin B12, vitamin A

1 large carrot, peeled and diced

100g (3½oz) boneless salmon fillet, skinned

1 tbsp whole milk or a suitable dairy-free formula milk for under 12 months or almond milk for over 12 months

15g (½oz) unsalted butter or dairy-free spread

2 good-sized ripe tomatoes, skinned (see tip, page 91), deseeded, and roughly chopped

30g (1oz) Cheddar cheese or dairy-free alternative, grated

For baby-led weaning, place the salmon on a piece of foil with a knob of butter, wrap up as a parcel, and bake at 180°C (350°F/gas 4) for about 15 minutes. Your baby can then eat the perfectly cooked pieces of salmon.

1 Steam the carrot for 15 minutes, or until tender.

2 Meanwhile, put the salmon in a small microwaveable dish, add the milk, cover with plastic wrap rolled back at one edge, and microwave for 1½ minutes, until the fish is just opaque. Leave to stand—it will continue cooking.

3 Melt the butter in a saucepan and sauté the tomatoes, stirring until pulpy (about 3 minutes). Remove from the heat and stir in the grated cheese until melted.

4 Flake the fish and mix this together with the tomato and cheese sauce and the steamed carrot. If your baby isn't ready for lumps yet, process the mixture in the food processor.

5 Freeze in individual portions. When needed, thaw overnight in the refrigerator or for 1–2 hours at room temperature, then microwave or reheat in a small pan until piping hot. Stir and allow to cool before serving.

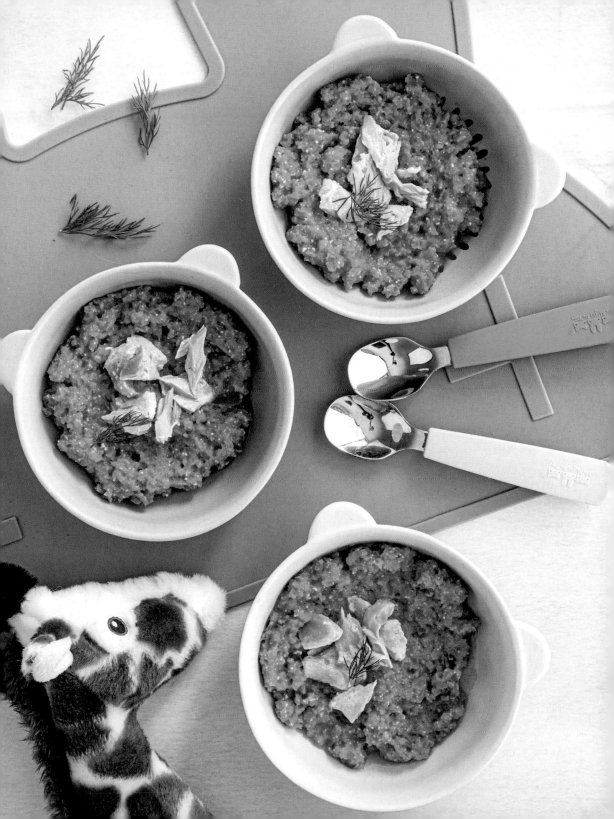

Ideally, you should give your baby fatty fish twice a week. A baby's brain triples in size during the first year and the omega-3s in fatty fish are very important for the development of your child's brain and vision. Try these tasty, power-packed salmon balls, which also have the advantage of being dairy-free.

SALMON, SQUASH, AND KALE BALLS

Suitable for freezing

Makes 20 • Suitable from 6 months • Prep time 15 minutes • Cooking time 15–18 minutes
• Provides calories, protein, vitamin D, vitamin A, omega-3 EFAs, vitamin K

50g (1¾oz) kale, trimmed
50g (1¾oz) fresh brown
   breadcrumbs or wheat- or
   gluten-free breadcrumbs
3 spring onions, chopped
1 tbsp freshly chopped dill
100g (3½oz) butternut
   squash, peeled and grated
250g (9oz) salmon fillet,
   skinned and diced
1 tbsp tomato ketchup
1 tsp soy sauce
Squeeze of fresh lemon juice

1 Preheat the oven to 200°C (400°F/gas 6). Line a baking sheet with nonstick paper.

2 Cook the kale in a pan of boiling water for 3 minutes. Drain and refresh under cold running water. Drain well and squeeze out the water. Roughly chop.

3 Place all the remaining ingredients in a food processor with the kale. Process until finely chopped. Don't add salt for babies under one year, but lightly season for toddlers over one.

4 Shape into 20 balls using wet hands and place on the baking tray. Bake for 12–15 minutes, until lightly golden and firm underneath. Alternatively, sauté in 2 tablespoons sunflower oil for 8–10 minutes, drain on paper towel, and leave to cool before serving.

5 Freeze in a plastic freezer container. When needed, thaw overnight in the refrigerator or leave out for a few hours at room temperature. Reheat in an oven preheated to 180°C (350°F/gas 4) for 10–12 minutes.

Flex it...

Use 2 tablespoons of snipped chives instead of the spring onions.

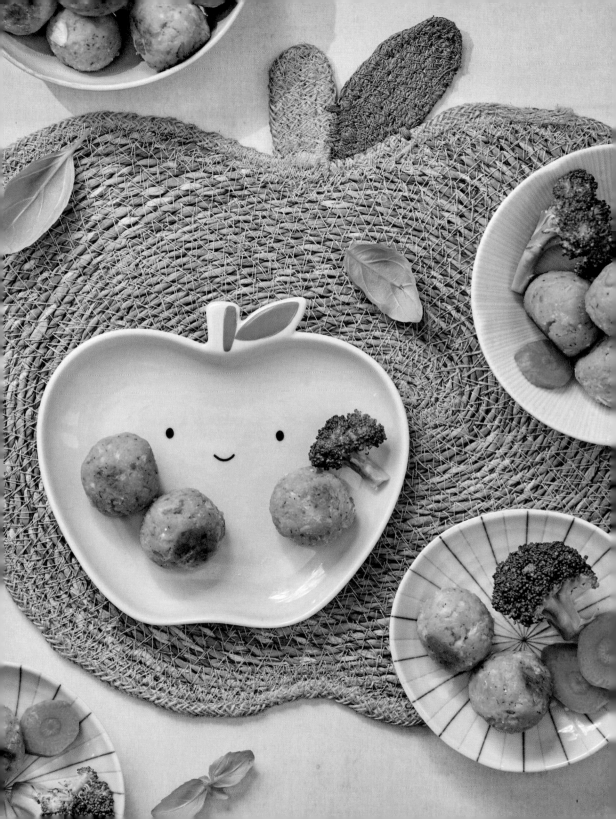

You will be amazed at some of the flavors that will appeal to your baby, so do introduce mild spices to add variety to her diet. Butternut squash is a fantastic source of beta-carotene, which your baby's body converts into vitamin A, essential for a developing vision and immune system.

MILD CHICKEN AND APRICOT CURRY

Suitable for freezing

Makes 3–4 portions • Suitable from 28 weeks • Prep time 10 minutes • Cooking time 17 minutes • Provides calories, fiber, protein, vitamin A, iron

1 tbsp sunflower oil
1 small onion, peeled and chopped
¼ tsp fresh ginger, grated (optional)
1½ tsp mild curry paste, such as Korma
100ml (3½fl oz) unsalted chicken stock or water
100ml (3½fl oz) coconut milk
4 dried apricots, roughly chopped
¼ small butternut squash, peeled and finely diced (about 150g/5½oz)
1 small chicken breast, cut into small cubes

For baby-led weaning, see the recipe on the opposite page.

1 Heat the oil in a saucepan. Add the onion and ginger, if using, and sauté gently, stirring for 5 minutes. Add the curry paste and fry, stirring for 30 seconds.

2 Add the remaining ingredients, bring to a boil, reduce heat, cover, and simmer for about 12 minutes, until the squash is tender and the chicken is cooked through.

3 Purée until smooth in a food processor or place in a bowl and use a hand-blender. For older babies, chop in a food processor or by hand to the desired consistency.

4 Freeze in individual portions. When needed, thaw overnight in the refrigerator or for 1–2 hours at room temperature, then microwave or reheat in a small pan until piping hot. Stir and allow to cool before serving.

EXPLORING NEW TASTES AND TEXTURES // STAGE TWO – 6 TO 9 MONTHS

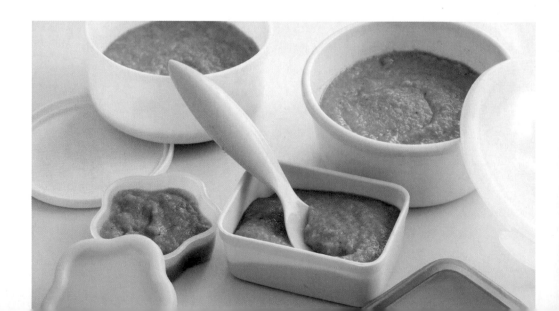

This is a great baby-led alternative to the curry on the opposite page. The mild fruitiness of the apricots and the creamy coconut milk add new flavors.

CHICKEN CURRY STRIPS WITH CURRY SAUCE

Not suitable for freezing

Makes 3 portions • Suitable from 28 weeks • Prep time 10 minutes • Cooking time 32 minutes • Provides calories, protein, vitamin A, fiber

1 tsp mild curry paste, such as Korma
1 tsp mango chutney
½ tsp sunflower oil
1 chicken breast, cut into strips

For the curry sauce

1 tbsp sunflower oil
1 small onion, chopped
½ apple, grated
¼ tsp ground ginger
1½ tsp mild curry paste, such as Korma
250ml (9fl oz) unsalted chicken stock
150ml (5fl oz) coconut milk
2 dried apricots, chopped
150g (5½oz) butternut squash, diced

1 Preheat the oven to 200°C (400°F/gas 6). Line a baking sheet with foil.

2 To make the curry sauce, heat the oil in a saucepan. Add the onion, apple, and ginger. Fry for 5 minutes over a medium heat. Add the curry paste and fry for 10 seconds. Add the stock, coconut milk, apricots, and butternut squash.

3 Bring to a boil, then cover and simmer for 15 minutes. Blend until smooth using a hand-blender.

4 Meanwhile, mix the curry paste, mango chutney, and oil together. Add the chicken and coat. Arrange on the baking sheet.

5 Bake the chicken in the preheated oven for 10–12 minutes, until browned and cooked through. Once cooled, serve with the curry sauce.

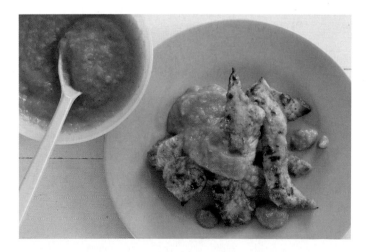

My son wasn't keen on eating chicken until I made mini chicken balls and added some grated apple. Even though he is now in his twenties, we still enjoy eating these Chicken and Apple Balls. These will be loved by the whole family.

CHICKEN AND APPLE BALLS

Suitable for freezing

Makes 25 • Suitable from 6 months • Prep time 15 minutes • Cooking time 25 minutes
• Provides calories, protein, iron, calcium

500g (1lb 2oz) boneless chicken thighs, diced

1 onion, diced

1 apple, peeled and grated

75g (2½oz) breadcrumbs or wheat- or gluten-free breadcrumbs

40g (1½oz) Parmesan cheese or dairy-free alternative, grated

1 tbsp freshly chopped sage or thyme

2 tbsp sunflower oil, for frying

1 Put the chicken into a food processor and process until finely chopped. Add the remaining ingredients, except the oil, and process again until finely chopped. Shape into 25 balls.

2 Heat 1 tablespoon of sunflower oil in a frying pan, add half the chicken balls, and fry over a medium heat for 5 minutes, until lightly golden on all sides and cooked through. Drain on paper towels. Add the remaining oil to the pan and cook the second batch of chicken balls in the same way.

3 Alternatively, preheat the oven to 180°C (350°F/gas 4). Arrange the chicken balls on a baking tray lined with nonstick paper and bake for 12–15 minutes.

4 Leave the balls to cool before serving.

5 Freeze in a plastic freezer box. When needed, thaw overnight in the refrigerator and reheat in the oven (see step 3).

Flex it...

Replace the chicken with the same amount of turkey or pork and the apple with the same amount of grated pear.

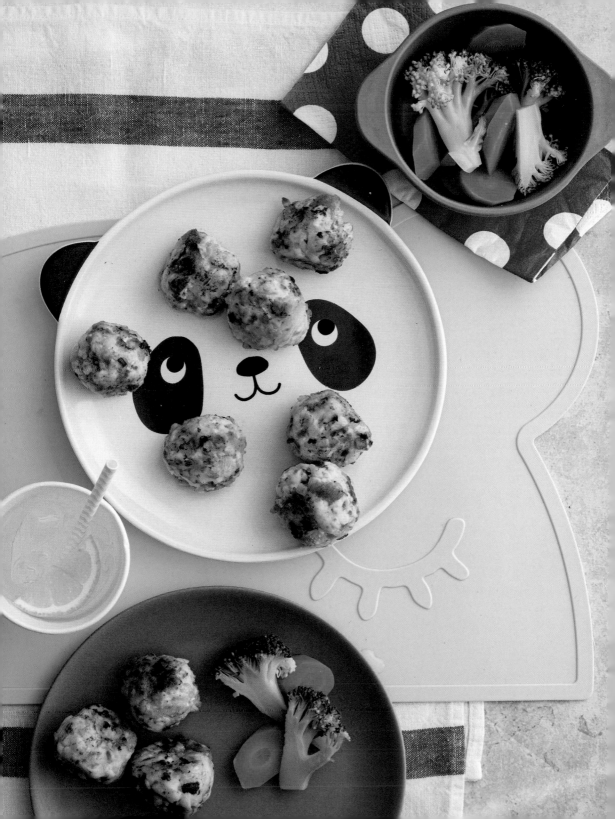

Children often eat with their eyes and you can add oodles of child appeal by shaping these into stars using cookie cutters.

CHICKEN, TOMATO, AND VEGGIE STARS

Suitable for freezing

Makes 4 portions • Suitable from 6 months • Prep time 15 minutes • Cooking time 15 minutes • Provides vitamin A, vitamin C, protein, iron and antioxidants

1 large banana shallot, peeled and chopped

100g (3½oz) Piccolo tomatoes, diced

1 tbsp freshly chopped thyme

250g (9oz) minced chicken

50g (1¾oz) Parmesan cheese or dairy-free alternative, grated

50g (1¾oz) panko breadcrumbs

1 tsp sundried tomato paste

1 Preheat the oven to 200°C (400°F/gas 6). Line a large baking sheet with a piece of nonstick paper.

2 Put the shallot, tomatoes, and thyme in a food processor. Quickly process for 3 seconds to roughly chop. Add the remaining ingredients and pulse for a few seconds until finely chopped.

3 Put a star cutter onto the baking sheet. Press the mixture into the cutter, then repeat with the remaining mixture, leaving a space between each star.

4 Bake for about 15 minutes until lightly golden and cooked through.

5 Freeze in a plastic freezer container. When needed, thaw overnight in the refrigerator or leave out for a few hours at room temperature. Reheat in an oven preheated to 180°C (350°F/gas 4) for about 12 minutes or until heated through.

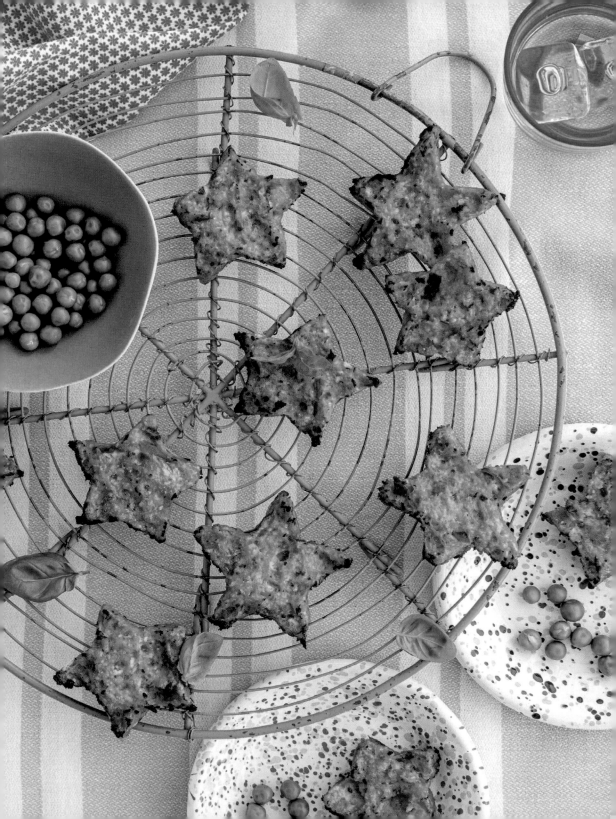

Chicken is often a firm favorite with babies, and it blends well with the soft consistency and mild fruitiness of puréed parsnip. If you wish, you can replace the chicken breast with boneless chicken thighs, which are higher in zinc and iron. This easy purée also freezes well.

CHICKEN AND PARSNIP PURÉE

Suitable for freezing

Makes 4 portions • Suitable from 6 months • Prep time 8 minutes • Cooking time 15 minutes • Provides protein, fiber, B vitamins, zinc

2 tsp sunflower oil

5cm (2in) piece of leek, sliced

1 small chicken breast, cut into small cubes

1 small parsnip, peeled and diced

85g (3oz) butternut squash, peeled and diced

½ small apple, peeled and grated

250ml (8fl oz) unsalted chicken stock or water

Good pinch of freshly chopped thyme or small pinch of dried thyme

For baby-led weaning, marinate the chicken for 15 minutes in a tablespoon of olive oil, ½ teaspoon chopped thyme, and ½ garlic clove, bashed. Then cut into strips and sauté for 2–3 minutes each side in 2 teaspoons of oil. Slice the parsnip into wedges, brush with oil, and bake in a preheated oven at 180°C (350°F/gas 4) for 20 minutes.

1 Heat the oil in a saucepan. Add the leek and sauté gently, stirring, for 3 minutes. Add the chicken and sauté for 2 minutes.

2 Add the remaining ingredients, bring to the boil, cover, reduce the heat, and simmer gently for 8–10 minutes, until all of the vegetables are soft and the chicken is cooked through.

3 Purée until smooth in a food processor or place in a bowl and use a hand-blender. For older babies, chop in a food processor or by hand to the desired consistency.

4 Freeze in individual portions. Thaw overnight in the refrigerator or for 1–2 hours at room temperature, then microwave or reheat in a small pan until piping hot. Alternatively, microwave from frozen. Stir and allow to cool before serving.

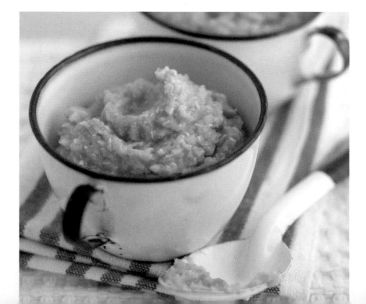

This is a delicious combination purée, and the addition of garlic and fresh basil works to bring out the natural flavors. It's also full of nutrients, such as vitamin A, fiber, protein, and antioxidants, to encourage healthy growth and development.

CHICKEN WITH SWEET POTATO, PEAS, AND BASIL

Suitable for freezing
Makes 5 portions • Suitable from 6 months • Prep time 6 minutes • Cooking time 20 minutes
• Provides calories, protein, fiber, iron, vitamin A, vitamin C

1½ tbsp olive oil
1 small onion, peeled and chopped
½ small red pepper, deseeded and diced
1 garlic clove, peeled and crushed
1 small chicken breast, cut into small cubes
2 tbsp pure apple juice
175ml (6fl oz) unsalted chicken stock or water
1 medium zucchini, diced
½ small sweet potato, peeled and diced (about 150g/5½oz)
4 tbsp frozen peas
6 fresh basil leaves, chopped

1 Heat the olive oil in a saucepan and sauté the onion and red pepper, stirring, for 4 minutes until softened. Add the garlic and sauté for 1 minute.

2 Stir in the chicken and continue to cook for 2–3 minutes, stirring. Pour over the apple juice and stock or water and stir in the zucchini and sweet potato. Bring to a boil, cover, reduce the heat, and simmer gently for 8 minutes. Stir in the peas and continue to cook for 3 minutes, until everything is tender and cooked through. Stir in the basil.

3 Purée in a food processor or place in a bowl and use a hand-blender. For older babies, chop in a food processor or by hand to the desired consistency.

4 Freeze in individual portions. When required, thaw overnight in the refrigerator or for 1–2 hours at room temperature, then microwave or reheat in a small pan until piping hot. Alternatively, microwave from frozen. Stir and allow to cool before serving.

For baby-led weaning, marinate strips of chicken in 1 tablespoon of olive oil, ½ teaspoon of chopped thyme, and ½ garlic clove, bashed, for 15 minutes. Remove from the marinade. Heat 2 teaspoons of sunflower oil in a frying pan and sauté for 2–3 minutes each side. Serve with roasted sweet potato: scrub the sweet potato, but don't peel it. Cut into wedges and arrange on a baking tray. Brush with a little oil and roast in a preheated oven for 20–25 minutes at 180°C (350°F/gas 4).

I like to add spices to baby food. Babies tend to eat well between 6 and 12 months and introducing a variety of flavors including spices like cumin and coriander will help avoid them becoming fussy eaters later on.

MILDLY SPICED CHICKEN WITH BUTTERNUT SQUASH

Suitable for freezing

Makes 4 portions • Suitable from 7 months • Prep time 7 minutes • Cooking time 33 minutes • Provides vitamin A, vitamin B, vitamin C, vitamin K, protein, fiber, iron, antioxidants

1 tbsp olive oil
100g (3½oz) red onion, peeled and chopped
3 carrots, peeled and diced
½ yellow pepper, cored, deseeded, and diced
1 garlic clove, peeled and crushed
150g (5½oz) chicken thighs, diced
120g (4¼oz) butternut squash, diced
4 dried apricots, chopped
½ tsp ground cumin
½ tsp ground coriander
300g (10½oz) canned chopped tomatoes
1 tbsp tomato purée
150ml (5fl oz) low-salt chicken stock

1 Heat the oil in a saucepan. Add the onion, carrots, yellow pepper, and garlic and fry for 2–3 minutes. Add the chicken, squash, apricots, and spices and fry until browned.

2 Add the tomatoes, tomato purée, and stock. Cover and simmer for 30 minutes until tender.

3 Blend to the desired consistency.

4 Freeze in individual portions. When needed, thaw overnight in the refrigerator or for 1–2 hours at room temperature, then microwave or reheat in a small pan until piping hot. Stir and allow to cool before serving.

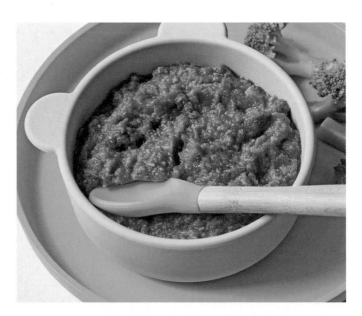

Red meat is your baby's best source of iron and she will love it cooked with apple and sweet-tasting root vegetables, such as sweet potato or parsnip. Some babies reject meat because of its texture; however, the sweet potato and apple in this recipe give the meat a nice smooth texture—not to mention a slightly sweet flavor that babies love.

BEEF CASSEROLE WITH SWEET POTATO

Suitable for freezing
Makes 4 portions • Suitable from 6 months • Prep time 12 minutes • Cooking time 1 hour 25 minutes • Provides calories, protein, fiber, iron, vitamin A, zinc

1 tbsp olive oil
1 small red onion, peeled and chopped
½ celery stick, strings removed and chopped
1 medium carrot, peeled and diced
1 garlic clove, peeled and crushed
115g (4oz) lean stewing steak, trimmed of fat and cut into small cubes
1 tbsp tomato purée
1 small sweet potato (about 250g/9oz), peeled and diced
1 small eating apple, peeled and chopped
1½ tsp freshly chopped thyme or ½ tsp dried thyme
250ml (8fl oz) unsalted chicken or vegetable stock or water
2 tbsp apple juice

1 Preheat the oven to 160°C (325°F/gas 3).

2 Heat the oil in a casserole and sauté the onion, celery, and carrot for 5 minutes, stirring until softened and lightly browned. Add the garlic and sauté for 1 minute, stirring.

3 Stir in the cubes of meat and sauté for 2–3 minutes until browned. Stir in the remaining ingredients. Bring to the boil then cover and cook in the oven for 1 hour. Stir halfway through. After 1 hour, remove the lid and continue to cook for another 15 minutes.

4 Purée until smooth in a food processor or place in a bowl and use a hand-blender. For older babies, chop in a food processor or by hand to the desired consistency.

5 Freeze in individual portions. When needed, thaw overnight in the refrigerator or for 1–2 hours at room temperature, then microwave or reheat in a small pan until piping hot. Stir and allow to cool before serving.

Beef is a good source of easily absorbed iron, which your baby needs for healthy growth, development, and optimum energy levels.

BEGINNER'S BEEF CASSEROLE

Suitable for freezing

Makes 5 portions • Suitable from 6 months • Prep time 10 minutes • Cooking time 1 hour 10 minutes
• Provides calories, protein, fiber, iron, vitamin A, zinc

1 tbsp olive oil
1 small onion, peeled and chopped
1 garlic clove, peeled and crushed
115g (4oz) lean stewing steak, trimmed of fat
  and cut into small cubes
1 large carrot, peeled and diced
1 large potato, peeled and diced
3 dried apricots, chopped
150ml (5fl oz) tomato purée
200–250ml (7–8fl oz) unsalted chicken or vegetable
  stock or water

For baby-led weaning, cut a small piece of steak into strips. Marinate in 1 tablespoon of olive oil, ½ teaspoon of freshly chopped thyme, and ½ garlic clove, bashed, for 10–15 minutes. Remove from the marinade and fry for about 2 minutes each side until cooked.

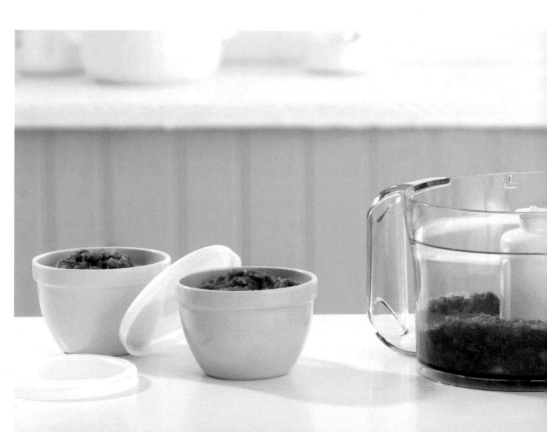

1 Heat the oil in a small flameproof casserole or heavy-based saucepan and sauté the onion gently for 3 minutes, stirring.

2 Add the garlic and sauté for 30 seconds. Add the stewing steak and sauté, stirring, until browned all over.

3 Add the carrot, potato, and dried apricots, and pour over the tomato purée and stock or water. Bring to a boil, stir well, reduce the heat as low as possible, cover, and simmer gently for about 1 hour, until the meat is tender, adding a little more stock or water if necessary and stirring occasionally.

4 Cool slightly, then purée in a food processor, or place in a bowl and use a hand-blender. For older babies chop by hand to the desired consistency.

5 Freeze in individual portions. When needed, thaw overnight in the refrigerator or for 1–2 hours at room temperature, then reheat until piping hot. Stir and allow to cool before serving.

BEGINNER'S BEEF CASSEROLE

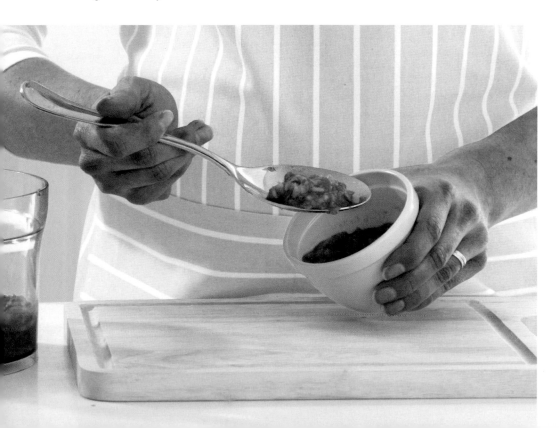

Simple and quick to make and the perfect summer finger food.
You can also make individual ones with blobs of yogurt piped
or spooned onto the baking sheet.

FROZEN YOGURT BARK

Suitable for freezing

Makes 12 portions • Suitable from 6 months • Prep time 5 minutes • Chilling time 3 hours • Provides vitamin C, fiber, folate, calcium, phosphorous, protein, fat, antioxidants

250g (9oz) full-fat vanilla yogurt or
   dairy-free alternative
100g (3½oz) strawberries, chopped
100g (3½oz) blueberries, chopped
50g (1¾oz) granola

1 Line a rimmed baking sheet with nonstick paper.

2 Pour the yogurt into the baking sheet and spread evenly so
   that it fills the sheet. Scatter over the chopped strawberries,
   blueberries, and granola. Place in the freezer until the
   yogurt is firm, about 3 hours.

3 Cut into 12 pieces and enjoy cold. Store the remainder
   in the freezer.

Flex it...

Put 150g (5½oz) blueberries into a
pitcher, add 1 tbsp water, and blend until
smooth using a hand-blender. Add the
blueberry purée to 250g (9oz) full-fat plain
yogurt (or a dairy-free alternative) together
with 1–2 tbsp maple syrup. Sprinkle over
150g (5½oz) chopped strawberries, 50g
(1¾oz) blueberries, and 50g (1¾oz)
granola. Freeze until firm and cut
into 12 pieces.

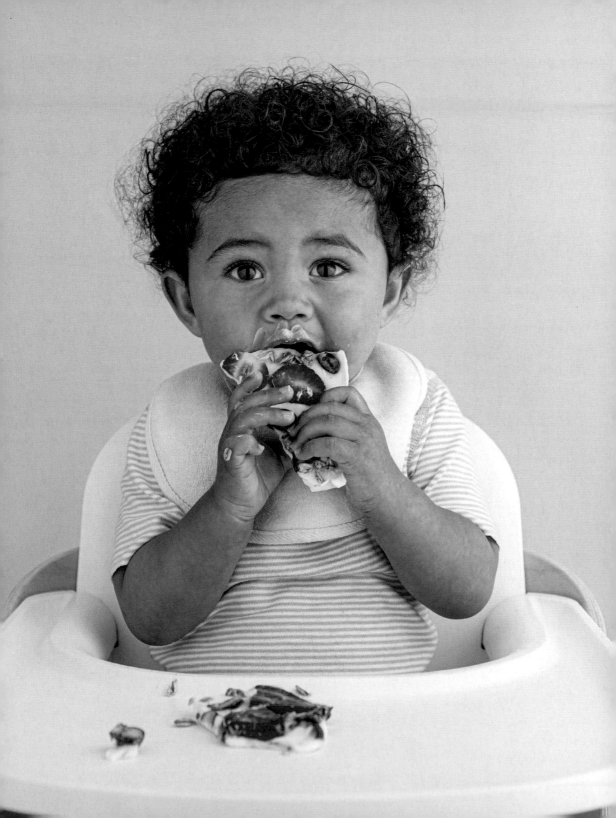

Always choose full-fat yogurt for babies and toddlers. Mix with gently sautéed ripe pears, cinnamon, and chopped apricots for natural sweetness.

PEAR AND YOGURT COMPÔTE

Suitable for freezing

Makes 2 portions • Suitable from 6 months • Prep time 3 minutes • Cooking time 2–3 minutes • Provides fiber, calcium, probiotics

Small knob of butter or
  dairy-free spread
1 large ripe pear, peeled and diced
1 tsp ground cinnamon, plus
  extra for sprinkling
100g (3½oz) plain yogurt or
  a dairy-free alternative
2 tbsp chopped apricots

1 Melt the butter in a saucepan. Add the pear and cinnamon and fry over medium heat for 2–3 minutes until the pear is soft and lightly golden. Set aside to cool.

2 Mash the pear with the back of a fork. Mix the mashed pear with the yogurt. Spoon into two small jars.

3 Sprinkle the tops with extra cinnamon and the apricots.

4 Freeze in individual portions. When needed, thaw overnight in the refrigerator or for 1–2 hours at room temperature.

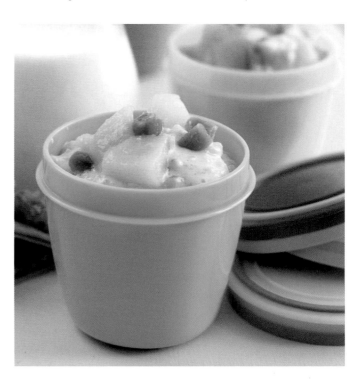

This planner is for when you have been able to progress to three meals a day. It's important that meals are made up of two courses to provide all the critical nutrients (see pages 13–15). In addition to the milk feeds shown, your baby may need a mid-morning and a night-time feed.

MENU PLANNER: 6/7 TO 9 MONTHS

Day	Early Morning	Breakfast	Lunch	Tea	Bedtime
1	Purple Porridge (p.82) with dates/stick of cheese/fruit	Sweet Potato and Kale Croquettes (p.86)/yogurt	Breast/bottle	Beginner's Beef Casserole (p.114)/fruit	Breast/bottle
2	Scrambled egg/ fingers of toast/ fruit	Poached Salmon with Carrots and Peas (p.95)/fruit/ yogurt	Breast/bottle	Tomato and Butternut Squash Pasta (p.92)/yogurt	Breast/bottle
3	Toast fingers with cream cheese or peanut butter/ fruit	Chicken and Apple Balls (p.106)/ broccoli/yogurt	Breast/bottle	Lentil Purée with Sweet Potato (p.91)/ Pear and Yogurt Compôte (p.118)	Breast/bottle
4	Iron-fortified cereal/fruit	Beef Casserole with Sweet Potato (p.113)/yogurt	Breast/bottle	Potato, Carrot, and Corn (p.84)/fruit	Breast/bottle
5	Iron-fortified cereal/fruit	Annabel's Tasty Salmon (p.100)/ fruit/yogurt	Breast/bottle	Mild Chicken and Apricot Curry (p.104)/ yogurt	Breast/bottle
6	Omelette or scrambled egg with whole wheat toast/fruit	Beginner's Beef Casserole (p.114)/ carrots/apple and plum with blueberries	Breast/bottle	Cod with Butternut Squash (p.96)/ fruit	Breast/bottle
7	Iron-fortified cereal/yogurt/ fruit	Yummy Rice with Butternut Squash (p.89)/fruit/yogurt	Breast/bottle	Sweet Potato with Broccoli and Peas (p.83)/yogurt	Breast/bottle

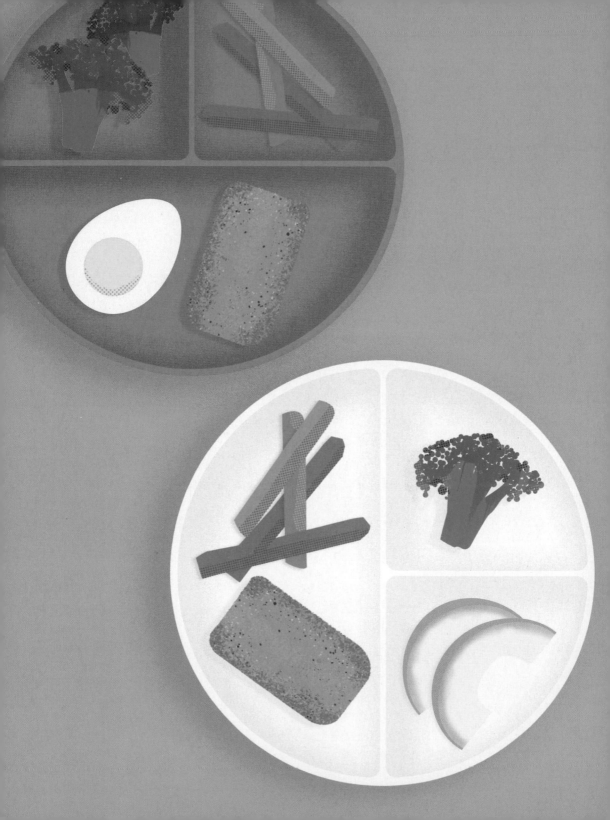

Creating a varied diet

Stage Three—9 to 12 months

Once your baby is happy with a variety of foods and textures, he'll become used to the idea of mealtimes and work toward eating three meals a day. As his milk intake decreases, it becomes increasingly important that his diet is balanced. You can adjust family meals to make them appropriate for his little tummy, and encourage him to eat along with the whole family.

• Menu planner page 156

A balanced diet

As your baby heads toward his first birthday, and you begin to give him fewer milk feeds, it becomes even more important that his diet is balanced and varied. His tummy is small, so everything he eats should contribute something to his overall nutritional intake.

How to plan your baby's diet

A balanced diet includes a variety of different foods. We know that babies need critical nutrients (see pages 13–15), and these are best provided through a varied diet. Offer a range of proteins such as pulses, fish, chicken, eggs, and yogurt. Wheat-based pastas or breads are a good source of carbohydrates, but include rice, potatoes, and different grains, too.

Experiment with fruit and vegetables, offering sweet potatoes and butternut squash in place of traditional favorites, and berries and exotic fruits, such as mango, instead of apples and bananas. Go for spring greens, spinach, or kale, and peppers and zucchini for color and key nutrients. The wider the range, the better.

Creating a balance

Including food from the four food groups helps to meet your baby's nutritional requirements:
- Potatoes, bread, rice, pasta, and other starchy carbohydrates
- Fruit and vegetables
- Beans, pulses, fish, eggs, meat; other proteins
- Dairy and alternatives.

Babies and toddlers eat smaller amounts of food than older children and adults, so it's important for them to eat regular meals and nutritious snacks. Babies need fat in their diet, so make sure that your little one is getting enough healthy fats (EFAs) (see page 14).

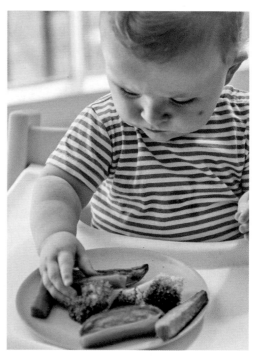

Five a day. Lightly steamed vegetables as a finger food snack help make sure your baby gets his five a day.

Three meals a day

At this stage your baby will be eating three meals and up to two snacks a day, although the amount actually eaten will vary. It's not unusual for one meal to be received better than the others, or perhaps your baby is a grazer, and that's fine, too. Don't forget, the purpose of weaning is to move away from milk and toward

Which food will your baby try today?

Aim for a good intake of critical nutrients.

food. Although your baby needs around 500ml (2 cups) of milk per day, it can be helpful for you to decide when you want him to have it rather than feeding on demand.

In the morning give him a little less milk so that he's more likely to eat a good breakfast, or if your baby is a late riser skip the early morning feed and give him milk at breakfast. You may choose to give him the rest of his milk feeds in between meals with a snack, or if it's easier give milk as a drink with meals instead of water, but don't offer this until he's at least halfway through his food, so that he doesn't fill up on milk.

Your baby will know when he is full. The professional advice now is not to encourage "one more spoonful" as this confuses a baby's built-in mechanism to self-regulate his appetite.

What can I offer for dessert?

By around 10 months, your baby's meals should consist of two courses—a main course and dessert or an appetizer and a main. This may

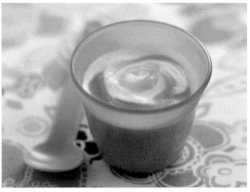

Time for pudding. Yogurt mixed with fruit purée, such as peach, is a healthier choice than ready-flavored yogurt.

sound decadent, but there is a scientific reason for it. An extra course offers your baby a new taste and texture and another opportunity to get those critical nutrients. Good dessert ideas are fresh fruit, yogurt, fresh-fruit ice lollipops (see page 155), or cheese sticks and breadsticks!

A BALANCED DIET

HEALTHY SNACKS

Snacks are another way of ensuring your baby gets adequate amounts of critical nutrients. At this stage, he should be having three small but nutritious snacks per day in between meals. Try to make sure that snacks contain at least two food items that contain the critical nutrients, one of which could be his milk. For example:

- Avocado on toast fingers
- Pita and hummus
- Fruit and a yogurt
- Chunks of cheese and breadsticks
- Peanut butter on rice cakes and milk
- Mini ice lolipops (page 155)

Moving on to new textures

Not all babies take kindly to lumps in their food, but most will master a variety of textures if you persevere. While it's perfectly fine to continue to purée some foods for your baby, by 9 to 12 months the time has come for her to learn to chew and swallow. The good news is that there's lots you can do to encourage her to enjoy expanding her food repertoire!

Mashing, mincing, and chopping

Mashing vegetables together, such as potato, carrot, and broccoli, with a little butter, milk, and grated cheese, is a good way to introduce different textures. You can also mash well-cooked and raw fruit, and it's a good way to blend several fruits and/or vegetables together without the use of your food processor. Mincing foods will also produce pieces that are whole enough to have a little bite, but soft enough to be chewed and swallowed easily. Once minced and mashed foods are accepted by your little one, try finely cutting and chopping her food, gradually increasing the size of the pieces as she becomes accustomed to the new texture. Some babies actually prefer larger, identifiable lumps to smaller ones that take them by surprise.

> **"While it's perfectly fine to continue to purée some foods for your baby, the time has come for her to learn to chew and swallow."**

Meat, poultry, and other proteins

Meat can sometimes be difficult for babies to chew, and this can put them off, so mixing cooked minced meat or chicken with pasta or mashed potato is good, or you can make mini meat or chicken balls or mini burgers. Pieces of roast chicken make good finger food. Alternatively, you can serve up breaded chicken or fish fingers. Tougher cuts of meat such as lamb and beef can be slow-cooked to make them more tender and easier to manage. You could also consider adding tiny pieces of meat to pastas and risottos, where they aren't quite so overwhelming.

Try offering healthy proteins, such as pulses, whole, in the form of finger foods. For example, chickpeas, lima beans, and even kidney beans are usually happily eaten by babies when you serve them this way.

Mixing textures

Create a little plate for your baby that offers foods of all sorts of textures. For example, you could cook some minced chicken balls, mash some potatoes, and offer some raw vegetables, such as carrot or cucumber, with a tasty dip. Or process together some cooked vegetables, such as carrots, zucchini, and sweet pepper, with a tomato sauce, and serve with pasta shapes, followed by a homemade cookie or mini muffin. You can also offer a variety of fruit, vegetables, meat, fish or poultry, dairy, and carbs at the same meal, allowing her to choose some from a tray of finger foods, and feeding her some of the smoother foods from a spoon. She'll end up

Mash, mince, grate, or chop!

Let your baby explore the textures with her hands.

chewing the finger foods at the same time as she takes in whatever you are offering on the spoon, blending the different flavors and textures. Encourage her to use her finger foods to dip and mush other foods on her plate. She'll be able to create her own concoctions, which will have a texture all of their own. It's good to have a plate or bowl with divisions, as babies like to keep different foods separate.

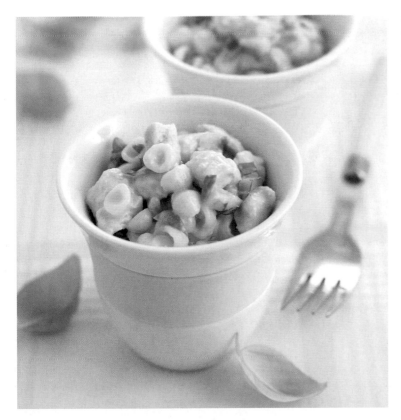

Chewing practice. Mix chicken bolognese with mini pasta shapes to help your baby get used to different textures.

Successful self-feeding

All babies will eventually learn to feed themselves and if you opted for baby-led weaning, your baby will have had plenty of practice already. You can encourage self-feeding by allowing your baby to experiment. Let him play with his food and make sure you give him plenty of finger foods to suck, gnaw, or actually eat, alongside every meal.

How long does it take?

Most little ones are unable to feed themselves properly using utensils before they are at least two or three years old, and until that time, they will rely on mom, dad, or their caregiver to make sure that the right amount of food makes it into their mouths. Your baby may object to you feeding him if he is feeling particularly independent, and you may have a tussle on your hands as you try to take charge again. You can, however, usually distract him in order to get a little food into his mouth, or help him guide his spoon in the right direction. Try to feed him a good proportion of his meal, so that you know exactly what he's getting. Although some babies can clear a bowl themselves in record time, chances are that most of its contents will end up in their bib, down the sides of their highchair, or scattered all over the floor.

Give your baby a small spoon or soft, flexible fork with a chubby handle that he can grip easily and allow him to scoop the contents of his bowl (or yours!) toward his mouth. Encourage him to pick up finger foods, too. Most things end up in a baby's mouth at this age, so it's a good habit to encourage, as he'll be more likely to try new things if he feels he's in the drivers seat.

He'll probably use his hands to eat even the messiest foods for many months to come, so be prepared by using bibs and putting a splash

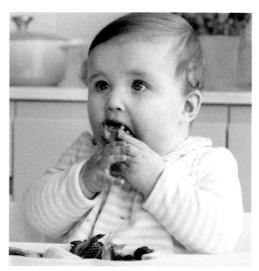

Touch and feel. Encouraging your baby to play with food is a key part of the weaning process, as she learns how to eat.

mat under the high chair so that food that is dropped on the floor can be recycled or more easily cleared up.

Playing with food

This is an important part of the developmental process of learning to eat, so it should be encouraged. The mess may be dispiriting, but your baby should be allowed to touch and feel his food, and to guide it in the direction of his mouth without fear of upsetting you.

He'll discover the way the different textures feel and taste, and will be interested in discovering new wonders.

Reluctant self-feeders

Some babies are simply not interested in feeding themselves and rely on you entirely to get food from bowl to mouth. While your baby is still very much dependent at this age and does require regular feeding alongside any self-feeding efforts, it is a good idea to encourage him to try. Why not buy a bright new set of utensils for him and give him a bowl that's all his own? Present it with a flourish and show him what to do. It's important to remember that babies are not born knowing how to use a spoon or fork, so you can guide his hand at every meal, or show him by doing it yourself, until he gets the hang of it.

> **"Let him play with his food and give him plenty of finger foods to suck, gnaw, or actually eat, alongside every meal."**

You may want to give him a bowl of food at the outset of his meal, when he's more hungry, and leave him to it for five minutes or so. Chances are he'll manage to get at least something into his mouth. Furthermore, babies are great mimics and like nothing better than being like mom and dad, or siblings. Give your baby plenty of opportunity to share mealtimes with the whole family, and he'll soon figure out what he's supposed to be doing.

If all the above fail, don't panic. Your baby may just enjoy the process of being fed and will get to grips with the basics later on. Continue to inspire him with delicious meals, and praise his efforts.

DAVID ASKS ...

My baby flings his bowl across the room and throws everything on his tray. I have no idea how much he's eating and the mess is driving me crazy!

First of all, you will need to accept that most babies are messy, and eating with their hands, playing with food, and mushing it between their fingers all encourage them to learn about different foods. In my experience, babies who are allowed to play with their food tend to be better eaters, because they enjoy mealtimes, have the opportunity to experiment, and learn to self-feed that much earlier.

Having said that, you can set a few basic ground rules. You can discourage him from throwing food by expressing your disapproval, and taking away his bowl each time he does this. You can also dispense with the bowl for the time being, placing his food directly on his tray, or investing in a bowl with a suction cup at the base to prevent it from being lifted.

You may also want to consider whether he's bored. Maybe he's had enough and wants to get out. Try removing the high chair tray and pulling him up to the table to eat with the rest of the family.

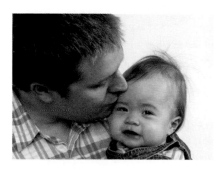

Family food

One of the best parts of introducing your baby to a greater variety of tastes and textures is that she can become included in family meals. Some recipes must be adjusted to make sure your baby isn't having too much sugar or salt, but this can make the whole family more aware of what's in their food.

Adapting family meals

Most whole, fresh foods are appropriate for babies and you'll simply need to be sure that you don't add salt or sugar (watch the condiments and cooking sauces, too). So, roasting a chicken, mashing some potatoes, and serving up some creamed spinach and baby carrots will provide the perfect meal for a little one. Finely chop, mash, or even purée the chicken and carrots and your child's meal is ready without further cooking. Similarly, you can process family soups, stews, casseroles, and even pasta dishes in your food processor for a moment or two, perhaps adding a little extra liquid to make it easier for your baby to manage.

> **"Sharing mealtimes helps create healthy, positive associations with food, as your baby learns to enjoy the social experience."**

What about herbs and spices?

Herbs are a delicious and nutritious addition to baby foods and can spice up, or make more fragrant, foods that might otherwise seem a little flavorless. Unlike salt and sugar, there are no specific spices or herbs that need to be off the menu for babies, but some babies simply do not like the taste of some flavorings and others may get upset tummies from some herbs or garlic. It's a good idea to try one new flavoring at a time and if there appears to be no problem, move on to try whatever your baby likes. Any of the green herbs, such as cilantro, basil, thyme, parsley, and dill, can be added easily, and you can use cinnamon, rosemary, and bay leaves while cooking fish, chicken, or vegetables. The more flavors to which your little one becomes accustomed while she's small, the wider the variety of "likes" that will be established.

If your baby likes the flavors and has no reactions after eating them (watch for diarrhea, crying, or rashes), then you can introduce whatever spices appeal. In some cultures, babies are brought up on strong, spicy foods and cope very well. So experiment to see what your baby will enjoy.

The importance of eating together

Sharing mealtimes helps create healthy, positive associations with food, as your baby learns to enjoy the social experience. Studies show that children who eat with their parents are more likely to consume more fruits and vegetables and eat fewer fatty and sugary foods. The reason is that they develop good habits based on the family ethos and also eat a wider range of foods, which they will try because everyone is eating them. Most babies love to copy parents and siblings, so offer your baby a little of your food and you'll be amazed by what she will eat.

Out and about

While it's a good idea to stay at home when you first start the weaning process, the time will quickly arrive when you'll need to feed your baby while you are out and about. You may also need to prepare meals for her to eat at nursery or daycare.

Transporting your baby's food
A good cool bag, with an ice pack, should keep your baby's purées at the right temperature. If you need to keep a purée chilled for a long period of time, you could invest in a wide-necked flask into which you can place some chilled purée or several frozen purée cubes. Make sure you heat the purée until piping hot and then let it cool before serving, to destroy any bacteria.

Many finger foods are easy to transport, and will last a few hours at room temperature. Fruit and vegetables, bread fingers, mini sandwiches, rice cakes, and dried fruits will all keep your baby's tummy full, no matter where you are. You can also choose foods that can be puréed, mashed, or cut into chunks on the spot, such as bananas, mango, papaya, or very ripe pears or peaches.

Your baby's lunchbox
Plan a lunchbox to include foods from the groups below. There should always be:
- Protein, such as meat, fish, tofu, eggs, hummus, yogurt, cheese, or beans
- Dairy, such as yogurt, cheese, or milk
- Fruit
- Vegetables or salad
- Carbohydrate, such as bread, crackers, couscous, pasta, or rice
- A drink—water or milk.

Note: it's fine to include a small lunchbox treat, such as a brownie, cookie, potato chips, popcorn, or pretzels.

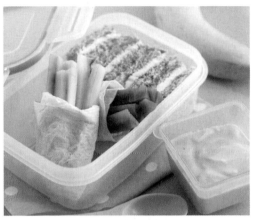

A taste of home. When you are heading out for the day, create a delicious lunchbox from your baby's favorite finger foods.

You can add child appeal by threading bite-sized pieces of fruit or veggies onto a straw or cutting sandwiches into shapes.

As your child gets older, involve her in making her own lunchbox healthy treats such as my Sweet Potato and Apple Mini Muffins (see page 151) or Egg-free Raisin and Oat Cookies (see page 152).

Eating out
If your baby is keen to try something from your plate, let her! While restaurant foods are likely to be high in salt or sugar, a tiny taste won't do any long-term damage and may encourage a sophisticated palate. Take a suitable weaning meal with you so she can eat alongside you.

Eggs are a powerhouse of nutrients. It's quick and easy to make mini frittatas simply by pouring the mix into a muffin pan, ideally a silicone one as then they are easy to remove once cooked.

FRITTATA MUFFINS

Suitable for freezing
Makes 12 • Suitable from 9 months • Prep time 7 minutes • Cooking time 40 minutes
• Provides calories, vitamin A, vitamin B6, vitamin C, vitamin D, vitamin K, calcium, protein, omega-3 fatty acids, antioxidants

Sunflower oil, for greasing
150g (5½oz) new potatoes
5 large eggs
75g (2½oz) Cheddar cheese or dairy-free alternative, grated
4 spring onions, chopped
6 cherry tomatoes, chopped
25g (1oz) fresh spinach, shredded

1 Preheat the oven to 200°C (400°F/gas 6). Grease a 12-hole silicone muffin tin or a metal tin.

2 Cook the new potatoes in boiling water for 12–15 minutes. Drain, cool, and cut into 1cm (½in) dice.

3 Beat the eggs in a large bowl. Stir in the diced potatoes, cheese, spring onions, tomatoes, and spinach. Pour the mixture into the hollows of the muffin tray.

4 Bake for 20–25 minutes until well risen and golden. Leave to cool for 5 minutes, then remove from the muffin pan and cool on a wire rack.

5 Freeze in a plastic freezer box. When needed, thaw overnight in the refrigerator and reheat in the oven for about 12 minutes.

Soft mini quesadillas cut into wedges or fingers make perfect finger food for your baby. Try this quick and easy nutritious filling.

PESTO AND AVOCADO QUESADILLAS

Not suitable for freezing
Makes 2 portions • Suitable from 7 months • Prep time 5 minutes • Cooking time 12 minutes
• Provides vitamin A, vitamin C, vitamin K, calcium, protein, healthy fats, iron, fiber, antioxidants

4 small wraps
2 tbsp fresh basil pesto
10 cherry tomatoes, sliced
½ large avocado, diced
50g (1¾oz) Cheddar cheese or dairy-free alternative, grated
2 tsp sunflower oil

1 Put two wraps on a board. Spread the surface of each with 1 tbsp pesto. Top with the tomatoes, avocado, and Cheddar. Put the remaining wraps on top and press down firmly.

2 Heat the oil in a large frying pan. Add a quesadilla and fry for 2–3 minutes on both sides until golden. Repeat with the next quesadilla, then slice into wedges to serve.

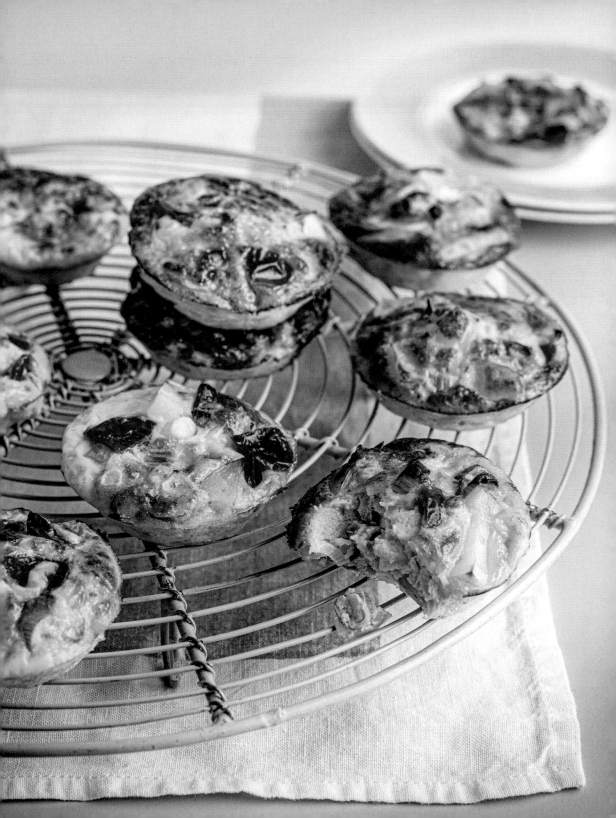

Stirring in fresh basil and Parmesan is a good way to add flavor as you can't season the delicious creamy tomato sauce used in this recipe with salt. You can freeze the sauce on its own in individual portions then reheat and add to freshly cooked pasta before serving if you prefer.

TOMATO AND BASIL PASTA

Suitable for freezing

Makes 4 portions • Suitable from 9 months • Prep time 5 minutes • Cooking time 20 minutes • Provides protein, fiber, calcium, calories

1 tbsp olive oil

½ small onion, peeled and chopped

½ garlic clove, peeled and crushed

1 small carrot, peeled and grated

200ml (7fl oz) tomato purée

3 tbsp water

2 fresh basil leaves, roughly chopped

1 tsp Parmesan cheese or dairy-free alternative, grated

1 tbsp full-fat cream cheese or dairy-free alternative

55g (2oz) conchigliette (baby pasta shells) or wheat- or gluten-free alternative

1 Heat the oil in a saucepan. Add the onion, garlic, and carrot, stir, cover, and cook gently for 5 minutes to soften.

2 Add the tomato purée and water. Bring to a boil, reduce the heat, cover, and simmer gently for 15 minutes.

3 Purée the sauce with the basil and cheeses in a food processor or place in a bowl and use a hand-blender.

4 Meanwhile, cook the pasta in a large saucepan of lightly salted water according to the package instructions. Leave out salt for babies under one. Drain and return to the pan. Stir in the sauce, cool slightly, and serve.

5 Freeze in individual portions. When needed, thaw overnight in the refrigerator or for 1–2 hours at room temperature, then microwave or reheat in a small pan until piping hot. Stir and allow to cool before serving.

Flex it...

Try grated celeriac or zucchini in place of the grated carrot.

As we don't add salt before one year, you need to find other ways to flavor food, like adding mild curry powder, garlic, and paprika. If making for babies over one, you could also add a little soy sauce.

VEGGIE FRIED RICE

Suitable for freezing
Makes 4 portions • Suitable from 9 months • Prep time 6 minutes • Cook time 9 minutes • Provides calories, B complex vitamins, vitamin K, fiber

1 tbsp sunflower oil
½ onion, peeled and chopped
1 small carrot, peeled and finely diced
½ small red pepper, finely diced
2 small garlic cloves, peeled and crushed
½ tsp paprika
1 tsp mild curry powder
250g (9oz) cooked long-grain rice
2 tbsp frozen peas
2 tbsp canned corn

1 Heat the oil in a frying pan. Add the onion, carrot, and pepper and fry for 5 minutes.

2 Add the garlic and spices and fry for 1 minute.

3 Add the rice, peas, and corn. Fry for 3 minutes.

4 Freeze in individual portions. When needed, thaw overnight in the refrigerator or leave out for a few hours at room temperature. Reheat in an oven preheated to 180°C (350°F/ gas 4) for about 12 minutes or until heated through.

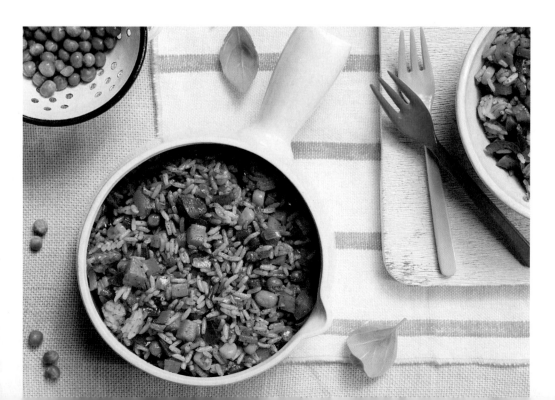

Just three ingredients make a surprisingly good pizza base and it's fun to get your little one to create pizza faces with their favorite toppings.

ANIMAL PIZZAS

....

Suitable for freezing

Makes 4 small pizzas • Suitable from 1 year • Prep time 20 minutes • Cooking time 35 minutes • Provides vitamin A, vitamin C, calcium, antioxidants

150g (5½oz) self-raising flour
1 tsp baking powder
125g (4½oz) Greek yogurt or dairy-free alternative

Toppings

2 tsp olive oil
1 small onion, peeled and finely chopped
1 garlic clove, peeled and crushed
400g (14oz) can chopped tomatoes
1 tbsp tomato purée
125g (4½oz) hard mozzarella cheese or dairy-free alternative, grated
8 cherry tomatoes, sliced
Handful of fresh basil leaves

Decoration (optional)

Stoned black olives
Chives
Mozzarella
Basil
Salami

1 Preheat the oven to 200°C (400°F/gas 6) and line a large baking sheet with nonstick paper.

2 Mix the flour, baking powder, and yogurt together in a large bowl. Gently knead into a soft dough. Divide into four pieces. Roll out to make four thin bases and place on the baking sheet.

3 Heat the oil in a saucepan. Add the onion and garlic and fry for 5 minutes until soft. Add the tomatoes and tomato purée. Simmer for 10 minutes.

4 Spread the tomato sauce evenly over the pizza bases. Cover with the grated mozzarella and scatter over the sliced cherry tomatoes and basil. Bake for 18–20 minutes. Decorate with the toppings of your choice.

5 Freeze in a plastic freezer box. When needed, thaw overnight in the refrigerator or leave out for a few hours at room temperature. Reheat in an oven preheated to 180°C (350°F/gas 4) for about 12 minutes or until heated through.

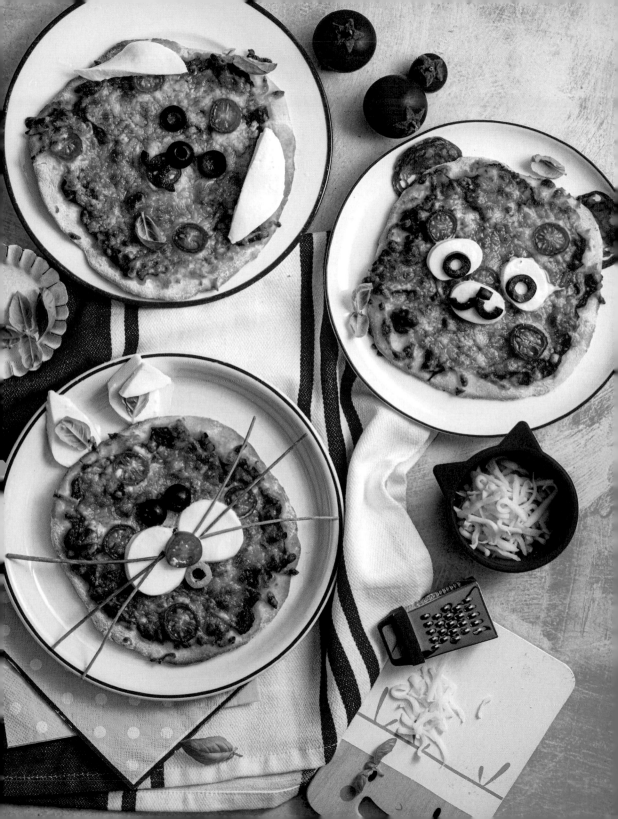

These individual fish pies are just the right size for your little one and perfect for freezing. Mixing carrot into the topping helps boost your child's five-a-day because potatoes don't count, but carrots do!

MINI FISH PIES

....

Suitable for freezing

Makes 6 portions • Suitable from 9 months • Prep time 15 minutes • Cooking time 35-40 minutes • Provides calories, protein, omega-3 EFAs, vitamin A, vitamin B12

40g (1½oz) butter or dairy-free spread

1 onion, chopped

1 tsp white wine vinegar

3 tbsp plain flour or gluten-free flour or 1 tbsp cornflour

150ml (5fl oz) fish stock

200ml (7fl oz) whole milk or a suitable dairy-free formula milk for under 12 months or almond milk for over 12 months

6 cherry tomatoes, quartered

1 tbsp freshly chopped dill

25g (¾oz) Parmesan cheese or dairy-free alternative, grated

450g (1lb) mixed salmon and cod, diced

Potato topping:

600g (1lb 5oz) white potato, peeled and diced

100g (3½oz) carrot, chopped

Generous knob of butter or dairy-free spread

1½ tbsp whole milk or a suitable dairy-free formula milk for under 12 months or almond milk for over 12 months

35g (1¼oz) Parmesan cheese or dairy-free alternative, grated

1 Melt the butter in a saucepan. Add the onion and fry for 5 minutes, then add the vinegar and stir until evaporated. Add the flour. If using cornflour, see step 2.

2 Add the fish stock and milk, bring to a boil and whisk until thickened. If using cornflour, mix it with 2 tablespoons of cold water and then add to the milk, and stir until thickened.

3 Add the tomatoes, dill, and Parmesan. Stir, then add the fish. Spoon into six ramekins about 10cm (4in) diameter.

4 Preheat the oven to 200°C (400°F/gas 6).

5 Cook the potatoes and carrot in a pan of boiling water until soft. Drain and mash with the butter, milk, and cheese. Spread on top of the pies.

6 Bake in the preheated oven for 20–25 minutes until bubbling. Allow to cool down before serving.

7 Freeze in individual portions. When needed, defrost overnight in the refrigerator or for several hours at room temperature. Reheat in an oven preheated to 180°C (350°F/gas 4) for 15 minutes.

Flex it...

Replace the cod with the same quantity of pollock.

In the potato topping, replace the carrot with swede, a nutritious vegetable that is high in vitamins A and C.

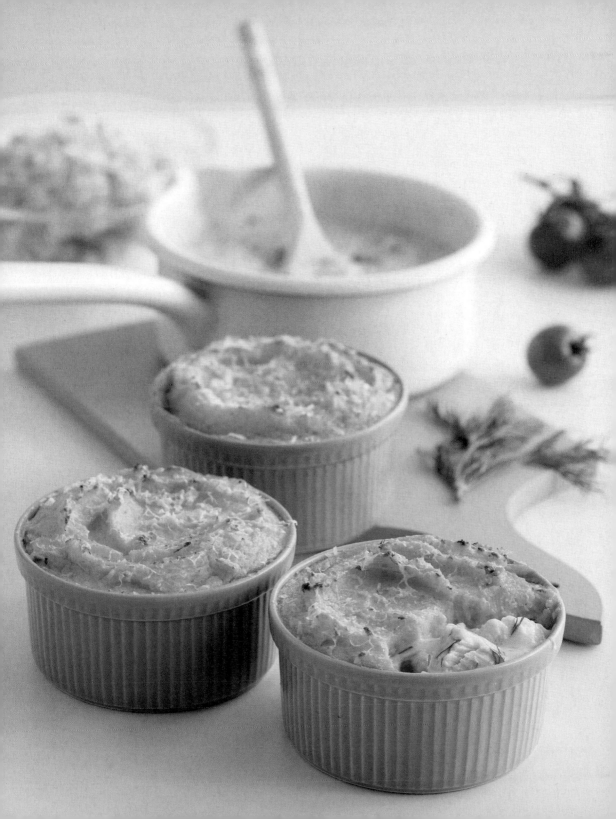

These delicious, golden fish fingers can be served to the whole family, and they provide plenty of good-quality protein. If you choose white-skinned fillets, there is no need to remove the skin. However, darker-skinned fillets should have their tougher skins removed before preparing.

FISH FINGERS

Suitable for freezing, uncooked

Makes 6–8 fingers, 3–4 portions • Suitable from 9 months • Prep time 10 minutes • Cooking time 4–6 minutes • Provides calories, protein, calcium, variety of minerals, B vitamins

75g (2½oz) fresh white breadcrumbs (3 medium slices bread) or wheat- or gluten-free breadcrumbs

20g (¾oz) Parmesan cheese or dairy-free alternative, freshly grated

2 tbsp roughly chopped parsley

Good pinch of paprika (optional)

2 fresh (not frozen) flat white boneless fish fillets (e.g. sole, plaice), about 100g (3½oz) each, skinned (see above)

2 tbsp plain flour or gluten-free flour

1 egg beaten with 1 tbsp water, or an egg replacement (see page 20)

Vegetable oil, for frying

1 Put the breadcrumbs, Parmesan, parsley, and paprika (if using) in a food processor and process together until the parsley is finely chopped. Transfer to a large plate.

2 Cut the fish fillets in halves lengthwise then into little strips.

3 Put the flour on a plate, and put the beaten egg and water in a shallow dish. Toss each piece of fish in the flour to dust, then dip in the egg, then roll in the breadcrumbs to coat.

4 If you are not cooking right away, put the coated fish on a baking sheet lined with plastic wrap, cover with a second sheet, and freeze for 2–3 hours until solid. When frozen transfer to a rigid container or sealed plastic bag and store in the freezer.

5 To cook, heat a thin layer of oil in a frying pan. Cook fresh or from frozen for about 2–3 minutes each side, until golden and cooked through. Drain on paper towels before serving.

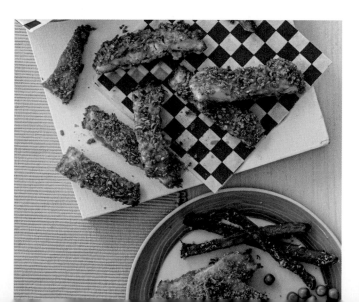

Did you know that from six months old babies should have fatty fish like salmon twice a week? I love this recipe as it's so easy—simply chop all the ingredients in a food processor and shape into mini burgers.

MINI SALMON BURGERS

Suitable for freezing

Makes 12 • Suitable from 9 months • Prep time 12 minutes • Cooking time 8 minutes • Provides vitamin A, vitamin C, vitamin K, calcium, iron, fiber, omega-3 fatty acids

250g (9oz) boneless salmon
   fillet, skinned
4 spring onions, chopped
75g (2½oz) carrots, peeled
   and grated
50g (1¾oz) Parmesan cheese or
   dairy-free alternative, grated
1 tbsp ketchup
30g (1oz) panko breadcrumbs
15g (½oz) kale, chopped
1 egg, beaten
Sunflower oil

1 Put all the ingredients, except the oil, into a food processor and process until finely chopped. Shape into 12 small burgers.

2 Heat a little oil in a frying pan. Add half the burgers and fry for 3–4 minutes until lightly golden and cooked through. Repeat with the remaining burgers.

3 For freezing instructions, see Annabel's Chicken Burgers (page 142).

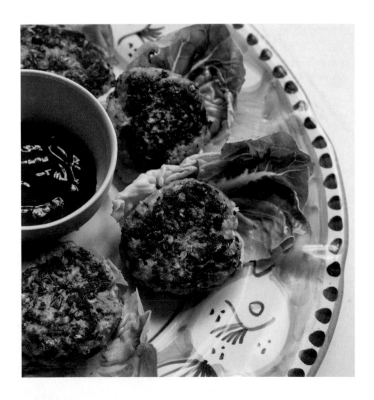

Sun-dried tomato paste is a favourite ingredient of mine but if you can't find it then you can blitz some soft sundried tomatoes in a blender. Tomato purée doesn't give the same flavor.

TOMATO, CHICKEN, AND RICE

Suitable for freezing

Makes 4 portions • Suitable from 9 months • Prep time 10 minutes • Cooking time 12 minutes • Provides calories, vitamin A, vitamin C, protein, fiber, iron, antioxidants

2 tbsp sunflower oil
1 onion, peeled and chopped
½ small red pepper, cored, deseeded, and diced
50g (1¾oz) butternut squash, peeled and diced
1 garlic clove, peeled and crushed
400g (14oz) can chopped tomatoes
1 tbsp sun-dried tomato paste
250g (9oz) cooked long-grain rice
100g (3½oz) cooked chicken, diced
1 tsp freshly chopped thyme
2 tbsp freshly chopped basil
50g (1¾oz) frozen peas
3 tbsp grated Parmesan cheese or dairy-free alternative

1 Heat the oil in a frying pan. Add the onion, pepper, and squash and cook for 4 minutes.

2 Add the garlic and fry for 30 seconds. Add the tomatoes and simmer for 5 minutes.

3 Add the sundried tomato paste, rice, chicken, herbs, and peas. Simmer for 2 minutes. Add the cheese.

4 Freeze in individual portions. When needed, thaw overnight in the refrigerators or leave out for a few hours at room temperature. Reheat in an oven preheated to 180°C (350°F/ gas 4) for about 12 minutes or until heated through.

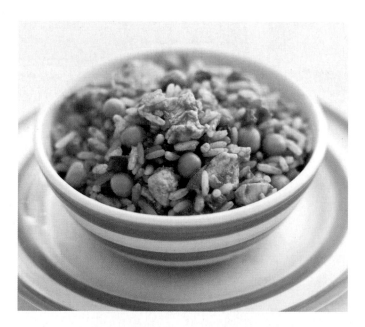

My cheat's cheese sauce is a simple mix of full-fat crème fraîche with Parmesan and Gruyère cheese. Frozen veg can be more nutritious than fresh as they are frozen within hours of being picked.

PASTA WITH CHICKEN, PEAS, AND TOMATOES

Suitable for freezing

Makes 4 portions • Suitable from 9 months • Prep time 10 minutes • Cooking time 14 minutes • Provides calories, B complex vitamins, vitamin A, vitamin C, vitamin K, protein, iron, calcium, antioxidants

100g (3½oz) pasta shapes
(e.g. elbow pasta or fusilli)
50g (1¾oz) frozen peas
100g (3½oz) chopped
cherry tomatoes
3 tbsp full-fat crème fraîche or
dairy-free alternative
100g (3½oz) cooked chicken, diced
50g (1¾oz) canned corn,
drained
20g (¾oz) Parmesan cheese or
dairy-free alternative, grated
20g (¾oz) Gruyère cheese or
dairy-free alternative, grated

1 Cook the pasta in a large saucepan of lightly salted water according to the package instructions. Leave out salt for babies under one. Add the peas 3 minutes before the end of the cooking time. Drain.

2. Put the tomatoes and crème fraîche into a frying pan and warm. Add the pasta, peas, chicken, and corn. Heat through. Turn off the heat and add the cheeses. Mix and serve at once.

3 Freeze in individual portions. When needed, thaw overnight in the refrigerator or leave out for a few hours at room temperature. Reheat in an oven preheated to 180°C (350°F/ gas 4) for about 12 minutes or until heated through.

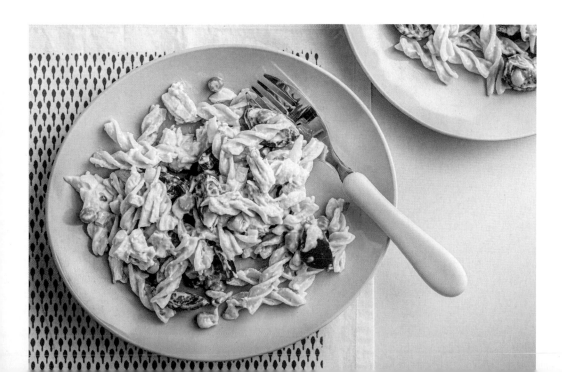

These soft, tasty burgers are bound to be a hit with your child—serve with steamed vegetables, such as carrots or broccoli, for a perfect balanced meal.

ANNABEL'S CHICKEN BURGERS

Suitable for freezing

Makes 24 mini burgers, 8 portions • Suitable from 9 months • Prep time 10 minutes • Cooking time 10 minutes • Provides protein, iron, zinc, calcium, B vitamins

2 tbsp olive oil

1 small onion, peeled and finely chopped

2 small garlic cloves, peeled and crushed

450g (1lb) minced chicken (mix of breast and thigh meat)

8 fresh sage leaves, chopped

1 eating apple, peeled and grated

40g (1½oz) fresh breadcrumbs (2 pieces of medium slice bread) or wheat- or gluten-free breadcrumbs

40g (1½oz) Parmesan cheese or dairy-free alternative, grated

Vegetable oil, for frying

1   Heat the olive oil in a small pan and sauté the onion and garlic gently, stirring, for 2 minutes. Allow to cool.

2   In a bowl, mix the chicken with the sage, apple, and breadcrumbs. Stir in the onion and garlic and the Parmesan.

3   Using your hands, shape the mixture into 24 small patties.

4   Heat a little vegetable oil in a frying pan and brown the burgers for 1–2 minutes each side. Turn down the heat to low and cook gently for about 5 minutes until cooked through. To test, push the point of a knife down through the center of one of the burgers. Hold for 5 seconds and remove. The blade should feel burning hot. If not, cook a little longer. Drain on paper towels.

5   To freeze, place the burgers (before or after cooking) on a baking sheet lined with plastic wrap, cover with a second sheet of plastic wrap, and freeze for 2–3 hours until solid. Pack in a rigid container or a sealed plastic bag. Defrost overnight in the refrigerator or for 2–3 hours at room temperature.

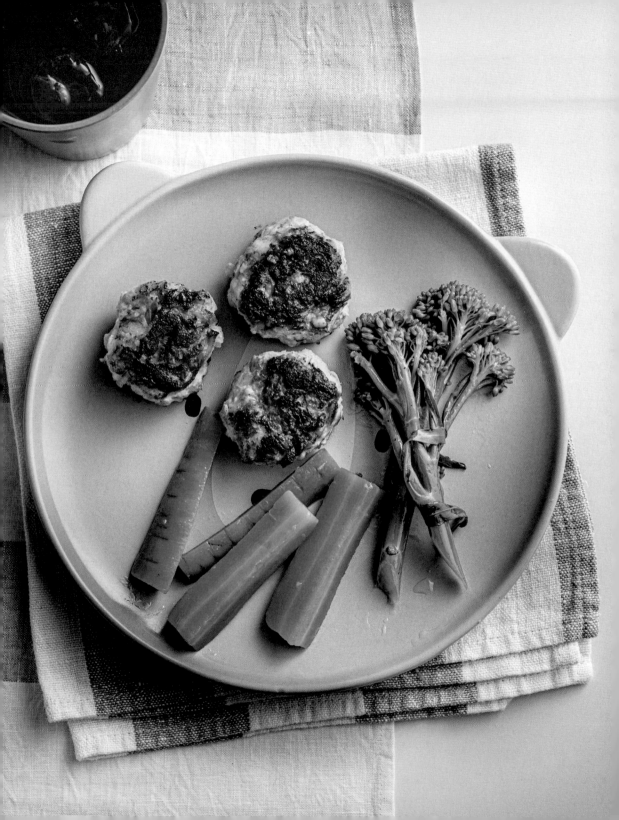

A very popular recipe with my children. I use minced chicken thigh, which has twice as much iron as the breast. The fresh thyme gives this recipe a delicious flavor but you could also use sage or a mix of thyme and sage.

CHICKEN BOLOGNESE

Suitable for freezing

Makes 4 portions • Suitable from 9 months • Prep time 8 minutes • Cooking time 35 minutes • Provides vitamin A, vitamin C, vitamin K, protein, fiber, iron, antioxidants

2 tbsp sunflower oil
100g (3½oz) onion, peeled and finely chopped
100g (3½oz) red pepper, finely chopped
2 garlic cloves, peeled and crushed
500g (1lb 2oz) minced chicken
100g (3½oz) carrots, peeled and grated
2 x 400g (14oz) cans chopped tomatoes
1 low-salt chicken stock cube, dissolved in 200ml (7fl oz) boiling water
1 tbsp low-salt soy sauce
1 tbsp tomato purée
2 tbsp freshly chopped parsley
1½ tbsp freshly chopped thyme
350g (12oz) pasta of choice

1 Heat the oil in a saucepan and sauté the onion and red pepper for 4 minutes. Add the garlic and sauté for 30 seconds. Add the minced chicken and stir until it changes color, breaking up any lumps with a fork.

2 Add the remaining ingredients, except the pasta. Bring to the boil, then simmer, uncovered, stirring occasionally, for 30 minutes.

3 Meanwhile, cook the pasta in a large saucepan of boiling water according to the package instructions. Drain and toss with the sauce.

4 Freeze in individual portions. When needed, thaw overnight in the refrigerator or leave out for a few hours at room temperature. Reheat in an oven preheated to 180°C (350°F/gas 4) for about 12 minutes or until heated through.

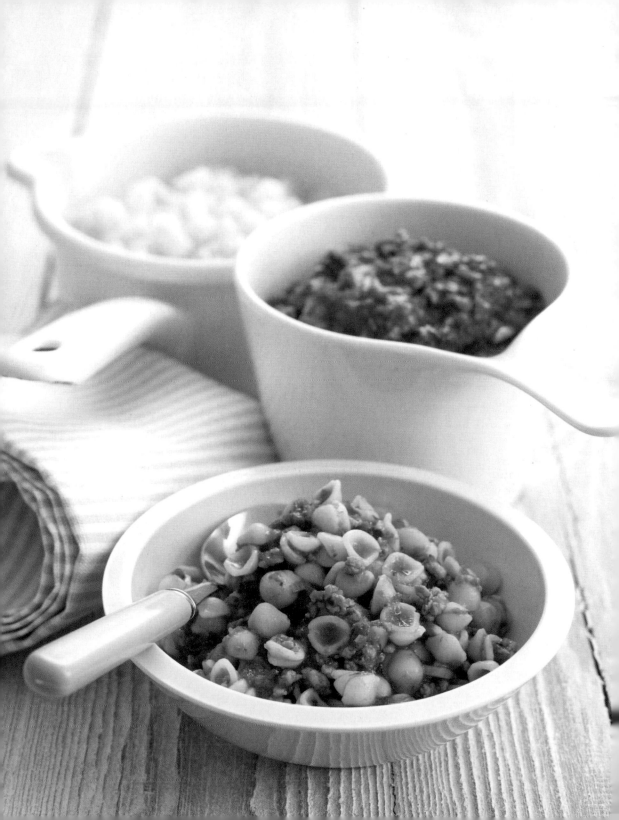

Made with baked sweet potato and cooked diced chicken, these delicious croquettes are the perfect size for little hands. They are deliciously soft and moist on the inside with a crispy golden coating. Serve with steamed veggies such as broccoli florets and mini carrots.

CHICKEN CROQUETTES

Suitable for freezing
Makes 8 • Suitable from 9 months • Prep time 15 minutes • Cooking time 10-35 minutes
• Provides calories, protein, vitamin A

1 small sweet potato
100g (3½oz) cooked chicken, diced
1 tsp chopped thyme leaves
2 spring onions, finely chopped
1–2 tsp soy sauce
1 tbsp sweet chili sauce
40g (1½oz) panko breadcrumbs or gluten-free breadcrumbs—half in the mixture and half to coat
1 tbsp sunflower oil, for mixture
2 tbsp sunflower oil, for frying
Salt (for over 12 months) and freshly ground black pepper

1 Prick the sweet potato. Bake in the microwave for 10 minutes until soft. Alternatively, cook the sweet potato in a preheated oven to 180°C (350°F/gas 4) for 30 minutes.

2 Leave the potato to cool, then scoop out the cold flesh—you will need about 100g (3½oz).

3 Place the potato in a bowl. Add the chicken, thyme, onions, sauces, 20g (¾oz) breadcrumbs, and the oil, and mix together. Lightly season, depending on your baby's age, and shape into eight little croquettes. Roll in the remaining 20g (¾oz) breadcrumbs.

4 Heat the oil in a frying pan. Add the croquettes and fry for about 5 minutes, until golden and crisp on all sides. Drain on paper towel and leave to cool before serving.

5 Freeze in a plastic freezer container. When needed, thaw overnight in the refrigerator or leave out for a few hours at room temperature. Reheat in an oven preheated to 180°C (350°F/gas 4) for 10–12 minutes.

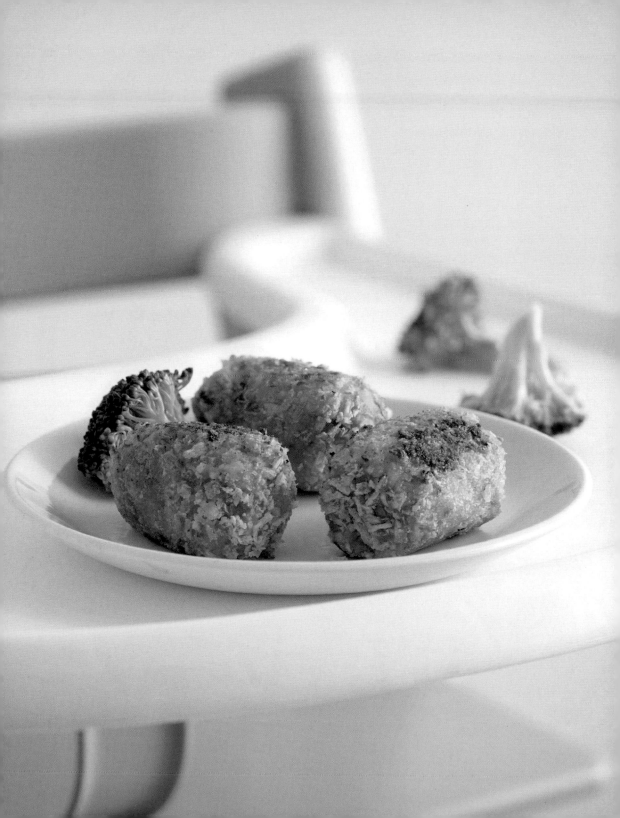

Who doesn't love a good bolognese? You can't go wrong with my favorite bolognese recipe with four veggies. You can freeze mini portions of bolognese in small ramekins mixed with pasta, rice, or top with mashed carrot and potato for a mini Shepherd's pie.

ANNABEL'S TASTY BOLOGNESE

Suitable for freezing

Makes 8 toddler portions or 4 adult portions • Suitable from 9 months • Prep time 10 minutes • Cooking time 30 minutes • Provides vitamin B, vitamin K, protein, fiber, iron, zinc

2 tbsp sunflower oil
100g (3½oz) red onion, peeled and finely diced
100g (3½oz) carrots, peeled and finely diced
100g (3½oz) red pepper, finely diced
75g (2½oz) celery, finely diced
2 garlic cloves, peeled and crushed
1 apple, peeled and grated
500g (1lb 2oz) minced beef
400ml (14fl oz) tomato purée
1½ tbsp freshly chopped thyme
150ml (5fl oz) beef or chicken stock (unsalted for babies under one)
400g (14oz) pasta of choice
3 tbsp grated Parmesan cheese or dairy-free alternative

1 Heat the oil in a saucepan and sauté the onion, carrots, red pepper, and celery for about 5 minutes. Add the garlic and sauté for 30 seconds. Stir in the grated apple and sauté for 1 minute.

2 Add the minced beef and sauté for 4–5 minutes until browned, breaking up with a fork.

3 Add the tomato purée and thyme and cook over a medium heat for 4 minutes. Stir in the stock and simmer for 12–15 minutes until the sauce is reduced and thickened.

4 Meanwhile, cook the pasta in a large saucepan of lightly salted water according to the package instructions. Leave out salt for babies under one. Drain.

5 Mix the bolognese sauce with the pasta. Serve with grated cheese or a dairy-free alternative.

6 Freeze in individual portions. When needed, thaw overnight in the refrigerator or leave out for a few hours at room temperature. Reheat in an oven preheated to 180°C (350°F/gas 4) for about 12 minutes or until heated through.

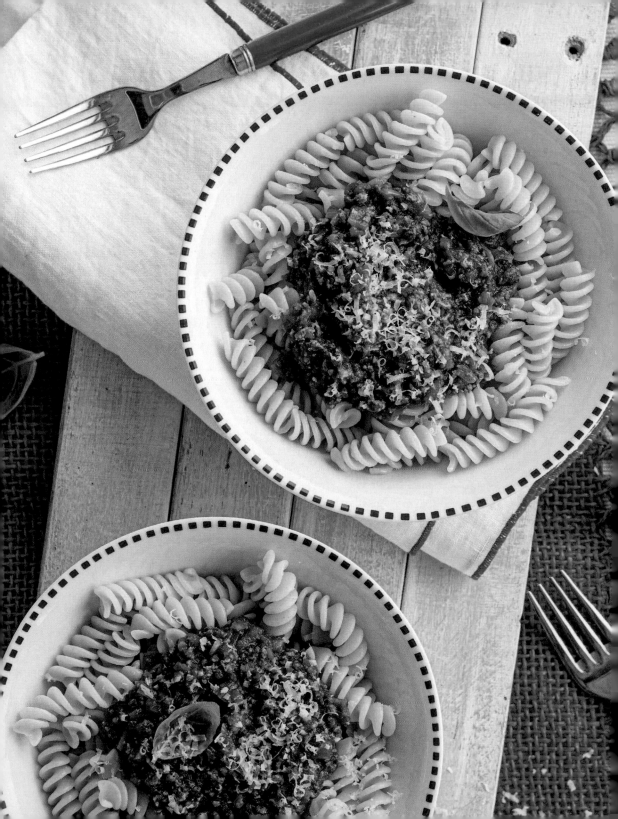

These tasty meatballs make perfect finger food on their own, but you can also serve them with the tomato and basil sauce used in the recipe on page 132.

MINI MEATBALLS

....

Suitable for freezing

Makes 25 mini balls, 6–8 portions • Suitable from 9 months • Prep time 15 minutes • Cooking time 10 minutes • Provides calories, protein, iron, zinc, calcium

2 tsp olive oil

1 medium onion, peeled and finely chopped

1 garlic clove, peeled and crushed

200g (7oz) lean minced beef

45g (1½oz) fresh white breadcrumbs or wheat- or gluten-free alternative

1 tbsp freshly chopped parsley

15g (½oz) Parmesan cheese, grated (see right)

1 tsp tomato purée

½ small eating apple, peeled and grated

¼ unsalted vegetable stock cube, crumbled

1 egg, beaten or egg replacement (see page 20)

Vegetable oil, for frying

1 Heat the oil in a saucepan and sauté the onion for 3 minutes, stirring, until softened. Add the garlic and sauté for 30 seconds. Set aside to cool.

2 Mix together the beef, breadcrumbs, parsley, Parmesan, tomato purée, apple, and stock cube. Stir in the sautéed onion and garlic, and add the beaten egg to bind.

3 Form the mixture into 25 mini meatballs. Heat the vegetable oil in a frying pan, and sauté until browned and cooked inside. Drain on paper towel.

4 To freeze, follow the instructions for freezing Annabel's Chicken Burgers on page 142.

For a dairy-free version, leave out the Parmesan cheese and add a beef stock cube.

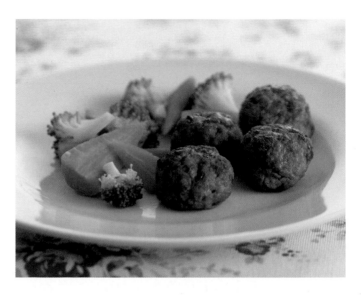

You can be a star baker with this foolproof and very yummy recipe.
These are good with sweet potato or carrot.

SWEET POTATO AND APPLE MINI MUFFINS

Suitable for freezing

Makes 12 • Suitable from 9 months • Prep time 10 minutes • Cooking time 18 minutes • Provides vitamin A, fiber, antioxidants

170g (6oz) self-raising flour
60g (2oz) superfine sugar
2 tsp baking powder
1 tsp ground cinnamon
1 tsp ground ginger
2 eggs, beaten
150g (5oz) sunflower oil
60g (2oz) maple syrup
1 apple, peeled and grated
100g (3½oz) sweet potato,
   peeled and grated
50g (1¾oz) raisins

1   Preheat the oven to 200°C (400°F/gas 6). Line a 12-hole mini muffin pan with muffin cups.

2   Measure the flour, superfine sugar, and baking powder into a bowl. Add the cinnamon and ginger.

3   Measure the eggs, oil, syrup, apple, and sweet potato into a bowl. Add the wet ingredients to the dry and mix well. Stir in the raisins. Spoon into the muffin cups.

4   Bake for 18 minutes until well risen and lightly golden.

5   Freeze in a plastic container with a lid. When needed, defrost at room temperature for several hours.

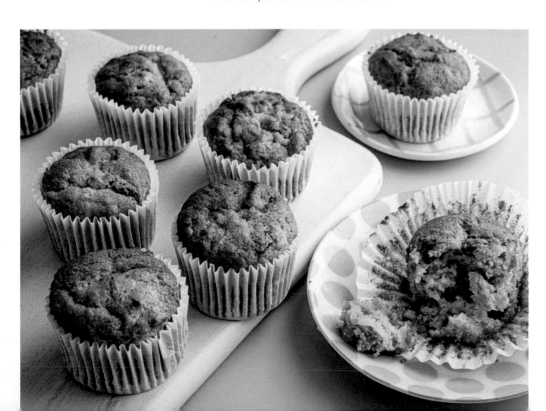

Did you know that the most common food to cause an allergy in babies is egg? We make this recipe all the time as it's easy, quick, and one of my favorite cookies.

EGG-FREE RAISIN AND OAT COOKIES

Suitable for freezing

Makes 15–16 • Suitable from 10 months • Prep time 10 minutes • Cooking time 12 minutes • Provides calories, fiber, iron, zinc

100g (3½oz) unsalted butter or
  dairy-free spread
65g (2¼oz) light brown sugar
1 tbsp golden syrup
90g (3¼oz) self-rising flour
½ tsp baking soda
Pinch of salt (if over 12 months)
90g (3¼oz) porridge oats
50g (1¾oz) raisins or sultanas

1 Preheat the oven to 180°C (350°F/gas 4) and line two baking sheets with nonstick paper.

2 Measure the butter, sugar, and syrup into a large mixing bowl and beat with an electric whisk until light and fluffy.

3 Stir in the remaining ingredients and beat again until the mixture comes together.

4 Measure into about 15–16 balls and arrange them on the baking sheets, leaving space between them to allow them to spread.

5 Press down to flatten and bake for 12 minutes.

6 Remove from the oven, leave to cool slightly, and then transfer to a wire rack.

7 Freeze in a plastic container with a lid. When needed, defrost at room temperature for several hours.

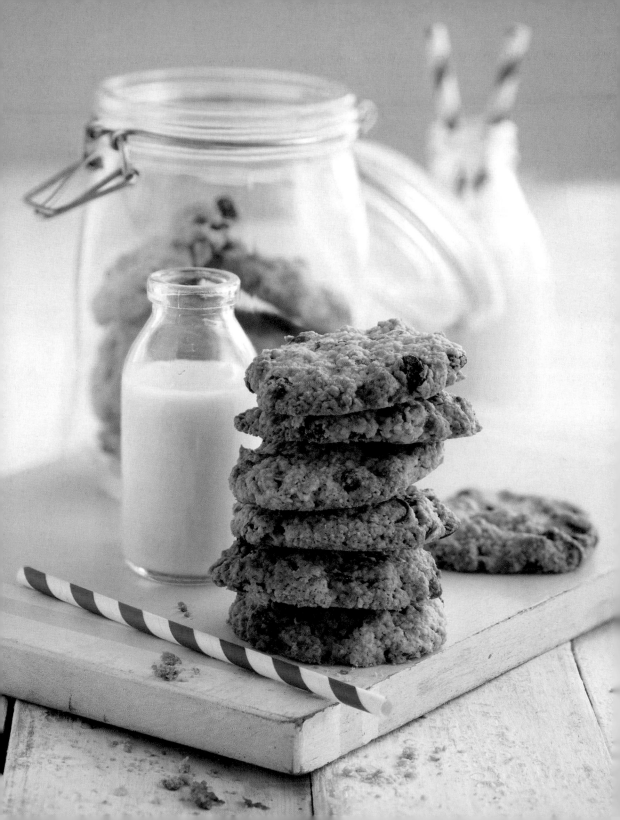

A no-cook treat that everyone will love, it's also a fun recipe to get your little one to help you prepare.

NO-COOK OAT AND CRISPY BARS

Suitable for freezing

Makes 16 • Suitable from 1 year • Prep time 8 minutes • Chilling time 1 hour • Provides vitamin A, vitamin C, vitamin E, calories, protein, fiber, iron, zinc, folic acid

100g (3½oz) unsalted butter or dairy-free spread
100g (3½oz) light brown sugar
100g (3½oz) golden syrup
150g (5½oz) porridge oats
40g (1½oz) puffed rice cereal
25g (1oz) pecans, chopped
50g (1¾oz) dried apricots, finely chopped
25g (1oz) dried cranberries
Pinch of salt (if over 12 months)

1 Line a 20cm (8in) square pan with plastic wrap or nonstick paper.

2 Measure the butter, sugar, and syrup into a large saucepan. Heat until melted.

3 Add the remaining ingredients. Mix well and spoon into the pan. Smooth the surface using the back of a spoon.

4 Cover and chill for 1 hour. Slice into 16 squares.

5 Freeze in a plastic container with a lid. When needed, defrost at room temperature for several hours.

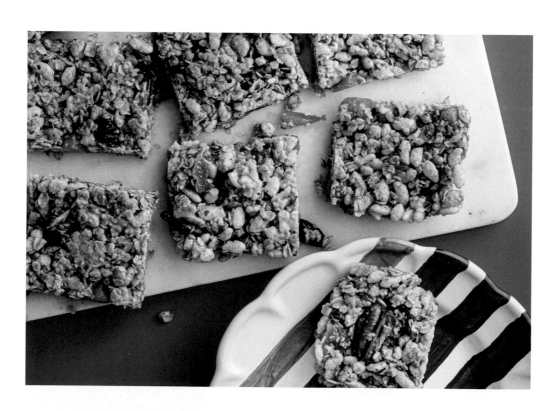

Ice lollipops are great for babies to suck on when they are teething. You could also make this lollipop using orange juice instead of tropical fruit juice.

TROPICAL BANANA LOLLIPOP

Makes 3–4 lollipops • Suitable from 9 months • Prep time 5 minutes • Provides calcium, potassium, vitamin C

½ small ripe banana
125g (4½oz) tub creamy
  vanilla full-fat yogurt or
  dairy-free alternative
100ml (3½fl oz) tropical
  fruit juice
1 tbsp confectioner's sugar or agave
  or maple syrup (optional)

1 Blend the banana and yogurt until smooth in a food processor or place in a bowl and use a hand-blender. Add the fruit juice and sugar or syrup, if using, and blend until combined.

2 Pour into molds and freeze for several hours or overnight.

Bursting with vitamins and minerals, these deliciously fresh lollipops are a perfect way to make sure your baby gets the nutrients she needs.

BLUEBERRY AND BANANA LOLLIPOP

Makes 4–5 lollipops • Suitable from 9 months • Prep time 5 minutes • Provides calcium, potassium, vitamin C

150g (5½oz) blueberries
6 tbsp creamy blueberry
  full-fat yogurt or
  dairy-free alternative
¼ ripe banana
1 tbsp confectioner's sugar or agave
  or maple syrup (optional)

1 Blend the ingredients together until smooth in a food processor or use a hand-blender.

2 Pass through a strainer to remove the seeds and skins (if preferred, but not absolutely necessary). Pour into molds and freeze overnight.

Tip: If you don't have ice lollipop containers, freeze the mixture in an icecube tray and stand a piece of plastic drinking straw up in the center of each for the "stick." Each mixture will make between 12 and 18 cubes.

Flex it...

Blueberries can be swapped for any other berry in season, or why not try a blend?

By now your baby will be eating the same foods as the rest of the family, albeit sometimes chopped. He'll also need a mid-morning and mid-afternoon snack (see page 123) and possibly an early-morning milk feed.

MENU PLANNER: 9 TO 12 MONTHS

Day	Early Morning	Breakfast	Lunch	Mid-afternoon	Bedtime
1	Frittata Muffins (p.130)/fruit	Annabel's Tasty Bolognese (p.148)/yogurt	Breast/bottle and snack	Fish Fingers (p.138)/ baked sweet potato wedges/fruit	Breast/bottle
2	Whole wheat toast with peanut butter/fruit	Annabel's Chicken Burgers (p.142)/ sweet potato wedges/fruit	Breast/bottle and snack	Salmon, Squash, and Kale Balls (p.102)/steamed vegetables/fruit	Breast/bottle
3	Purple Porridge (p.82) with dates/fruit	Mini Meatballs (p.150)/steamed broccoli and carrots/ Fruit Lollipop (p.155)	Breast/bottle and snack	Chicken and Apple Balls (p.106)/fruit	Breast/bottle
4	Scrambled egg and toast fingers/fruit	Mini Salmon Burgers (p.139)/dried apricots and fresh pear	Breast/bottle and snack	Veggie Fried Rice (p.133)/No-cook Oat and Crispy Bars (p.154)	Breast/bottle
5	Granola, fruit, and yogurt/ cheese	Annabel's Chicken Burgers (p.142)/bun, avocado, and red pepper/yogurt	Breast/bottle and snack	Mini Meatballs (p.150)/pasta/ carrots/ broccoli/fruit	Breast/bottle
6	Boiled egg with soldiers/ fruit	Chicken Croquettes (p.146)/carrot sticks/ Raisin and Oat Cookies (p.152)	Breast/bottle and snack	Mini Fish Pies (p.136)/fruit	Breast/bottle
7	Iron-fortified breakfast cereal/yogurt/ fruit sticks	Sweet Potato and Kale Croquettes (p.86)/Fruit lollipops (p.155)	Breast/bottle and snack	Annabel's Tasty Bolognese (p.148)/steamed vegetables/fruit	Breast/bottle

ABOUT ANNABEL KARMEL, MBE

Over 30 years of recipes and expert advice

With expertise spanning over 30 years, mother of three Annabel Karmel reigns as the UK's no. 1 children's cookbook author, bestselling international author, and a world-leading expert on devising delicious, nutritious meals for babies, children, and families.

Since launching her revolutionary cookbook for babies—The Complete Baby and Toddler Meal Planner—in 1991, a feeding "bible" that has sold over 6 million copies and become the second bestselling nonfiction hardback of all time, Annabel has raised millions of families on her recipes. With more than 50 cookbooks published, Annabel's vision has always been to ensure that every child gets the nutrition they need for their development and long-term health. Navigating a world of food for babies can be overwhelming, so Annabel simplifies that all-important journey with tried and tested recipes and the latest researched advice.

If you haven't joined already, check out Annabel's social media community for even more recipes, ideas, and support. Her award-winning Baby & Toddler Recipe App is also jam-packed with 700+ recipes and lots of helpful features.

In 2006, Annabel received an MBE in the Queen's Birthday Honours for her outstanding work in the field of child nutrition. From kitchen table to global stage, Annabel is loved and trusted all over the world for raising healthy, happy eaters.

Scan for recipe app & lots more!

www.annabelkarmel.com   Instagram: annabelkarmel   Facebook: annabelkarmeluk

Thanks to Bugaboo for providing their clever Bugaboo Giraffe chairs for this book. From newborns to toddlers and beyond, the beautifully designed eco-friendly chair is super versatile as your child grows.

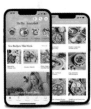

Award-winning recipe app

ACKNOWLEDGMENTS

First Edition

DK UK

Project editor Helen Murray
Editorial assistance Angela Baynham
Designer Jo Grey
Senior art editor Sara Kimmins
Jacket designer and design assistant Charlotte Seymour
Managing editor Penny Warren
Managing art editors Glenda Fisher and Marianne Markham
Senior production editor Jennifer Murray
Production controller Hema Gohil
Creative technical support Sonia Charbonnier
Category publisher Peggy Vance
Editorial consultant Karen Sullivan
Allergy consultant Dr. Adam Fox
Nutritional consultant Dr. Rosan Meyer
Food styling Seiko Hatfield
Home economist Carolyn Humphries
Photographer Dave King
Photography art direction Peggy Sadler

Third Edition

Author's Acknowledgments

Special thanks to the wonderful team involved in producing this book: Cara Armstrong, Jasmin Lennie, Mary-Clare Jerram, Lucinda McCord, Jonathan Lloyd, Peggy Vance, Ant Duncan, Emily Carter, Lucy Drayson, and Sarah Smith.

Publisher's Acknowledgments

Dorling Kindersley UK would like to thank Eleanor Ridsdale for jacket design and spread styling; Ant Duncan for new photography; Lizzie Evans for food styling; Charlie Phillips for prop styling; Vicky Orchard for editing; Kathy Steer for proofreading; and Hilary Bird for indexing.

Picture Credits

The publisher would like to thank Annabel Karmel for her kind permission to reproduce the photographs for the following pages: 1, 7, 26, 31, 85, 101, 107, 109, 135, 138, 141, 149, 153 (Ant Duncan); 11, 88, 91, 103, 112, 122 (Greg Woodward); 14, 48, 72, 82, 89, 110, 118, 140, 145 (Dave King); 77, 133, 139 (Emily Carter); 80, 126 (Tia Tallula).

All other images © Dorling Kindersley. For further information see: www.dkimages.com

Index

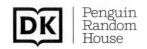

Weaning resources

CENTERS FOR DISEASE CONTROL AND PREVENTION (CDC) /WEANING/ NUTRITION
www.cdc.gov

AMERICAN ACADEMY OF PEDIATRICS INFANT FOOD AND FEEDING
www.aap.org/en/patient-care/healthy-active-living-for-families/infant-food-and-feeding/

Allergy

AMERICAN COLLEGE OF ALLERGY, ASTHMA, AND IMMUNOLOGY
www.acaai.org

LIVING WITH FOOD ALLERGIES
www.foodallergy.org

Breastfeeding

USDA WIC BREASTFEEDING SUPPORT
www.wicbreastfeeding.fns.usda.gov

US BREASTFEEDING COMMITTEE (USBC)
www.usbreastfeeding.org

LA LECHE LEAGUE USA
www.lllusa.org

Nutrition and health

ACADEMY OF NUTRITION AND DIETETICS
www.eatright.org

AMERICAN NUTRITION ASSOCIATION
theana.org

FOOD STANDARDS AGENCY
www.foodsafety.gov

AMERICAN VEGAN SOCIETY
americanvegan.org

NORTH AMERICAN VEGETARIAN SOCIETY (NAVS)
navs-online.org

DK LONDON
Editorial Director Cara Armstrong
Assistant Editor Jasmin Lennie
US Editor Jill Hamilton
US Consultant Ginger Hultin, MS, RDN
Senior Designer Glenda Fisher
Production Editor Tony Phipps
Production Controller Stephanie McConnell
Art Director Maxine Pedliham
Publishing Director Katie Cowan

Jacket Designer Eleanor Ridsdale
Photographer Ant Duncan

DK INDIA
Managing Art Editor Neha Ahuja Chowdhry
DTP Designers Manish Upreti and Satish Gaur
DTP Coordinator Pushpak Tyagi
Pre-production Manager Balwant Singh
Creative Head Malavika Talukder

This American Edition, 2024
First American Edition, 2015
Published in the United States by DK Publishing
1745 Broadway, 20th Floor, New York, NY 10019

Copyright © 2015, 2018, 2024 Dorling Kindersley Limited
DK, a Division of Penguin Random House LLC
24 25 26 27 28   10 9 8 7 6 5 4 3 2
002–339054–May/2024

A catalog record for this book
is available from the Library of Congress.
ISBN 978-0-7440-9291-2

DK books are available at special discounts when purchased in bulk for sales promotions, premiums, fund-raising, or educational use. For details, contact: DK Publishing Special Markets,
1745 Broadway, 20th Floor, New York, NY 10019
SpecialSales@dk.com
Printed and bound in China

www.dk.com

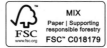

MIX
Paper | Supporting
responsible forestry
FSC™ C018179

This book was made with Forest Stewardship Council™ certified paper - one small step in DK's commitment to a sustainable future.
For more information go to www.dk.com/our-green-pledge